The Achalasia Mastery Bible: Your Blueprint for Complete Achalasia Management

Dr. Ankita Kashyap and Prof. Krishna N. Sharma

Published by Virtued Press, 2023.

While every precaution has been taken in the preparation of this book, the publisher assumes no responsibility for errors or omissions, or for damages resulting from the use of the information contained herein.

THE ACHALASIA MASTERY BIBLE: YOUR BLUEPRINT FOR COMPLETE ACHALASIA MANAGEMENT

First edition. December 29, 2023.

Copyright © 2023 Dr. Ankita Kashyap and Prof. Krishna N. Sharma.

ISBN: 979-8215066447

Written by Dr. Ankita Kashyap and Prof. Krishna N. Sharma.

Table of Contents

....	1
Introduction	2
Understanding Achalasia	5
The Dawn of Discovery: Achalasia's History	6
Defining Achalasia: More Than Just a Word	9
Anatomy of the Esophagus: A Critical Pipeline	15
A Closer Look at the Lower Esophageal Sphincter	18
The Symptoms Spectrum: From Mild to Severe	23
The Psychological Impact of Achalasia	27
Epidemiology: Understanding the Statistics	29
Diagnosis and Assessment	35
Recognizing the Signs: When to Seek Help	36
The Role of the Primary Care Physician	39
Advanced Diagnostic Techniques	45
Misdiagnosis: Common Pitfalls and Prevention	49
The Patient's Role in Diagnosis	53
Interpreting Test Results: A Guide for Patients	56
Case Study: A Diagnostic Journey	60
Treatment Options	63
Pharmacological Interventions: Medications and Beyond ...	64
Endoscopic Procedures: A Minimally Invasive Approach ...	66
Surgical Solutions: When to Consider	71
Botox Injections: A Temporary Relief	75
The Role of Diet in Managing Symptoms	79
Emerging Therapies: Future of Achalasia Treatment	82
Choosing the Right Treatment: A Personalized Approach ...	85
Meal Planning and Preparation: Strategies for Success ..	87
Eating Techniques: Minimizing Discomfort	93
The Impact of Exercise on Achalasia	97
Stress Management and Achalasia	100
Navigating Social Situations With Achalasia	103

Vitamins and Supplements: Are They Helpful? 107
Mind-Body Techniques: A Path to Inner Balance 110
Chiropractic Care: Aligning for Health 112
Homeopathy and Achalasia: A Diluted Solution? 116
Massage Therapy: Easing the Esophageal Tension 120
Energy Healing: Beyond the Physical Realm 126
Mental Health and Emotional Well-being 132
Coping With Chronic Illness: Achalasia's Mental Toll 133
Therapy Options: Talking It Out 136
Mindfulness and Meditation: Finding Peace Amidst Pain 142
The Role of Family and Friends: A Support Network 145
Navigating Depression and Anxiety 150
Self-help Techniques for Emotional Regulation 153
Personal Stories: Triumphs Over Achalasia 156
The Future of Achalasia Research 159
Clinical Trials: The Frontier of Achalasia Treatment 160
Genetic Research: Unraveling the DNA of Achalasia 164
The Quest for a Cure: How Close Are We? 167
Innovations in Diagnostic Technology 170
Patient Advocacy and Awareness Campaigns 173
The Role of Artificial Intelligence in Achalasia 178
Global Collaboration in Achalasia Research 181

Table of Contents

....	1
Introduction	2
Understanding Achalasia	5
The Dawn of Discovery: Achalasia's History	6
Defining Achalasia: More Than Just a Word	9
Anatomy of the Esophagus: A Critical Pipeline	15
A Closer Look at the Lower Esophageal Sphincter	18
The Symptoms Spectrum: From Mild to Severe	23
The Psychological Impact of Achalasia	27
Epidemiology: Understanding the Statistics	29
Diagnosis and Assessment	35
Recognizing the Signs: When to Seek Help	36
The Role of the Primary Care Physician	39
Advanced Diagnostic Techniques	45
Misdiagnosis: Common Pitfalls and Prevention	49
The Patient's Role in Diagnosis	53
Interpreting Test Results: A Guide for Patients	56
Case Study: A Diagnostic Journey	60
Treatment Options	63
Pharmacological Interventions: Medications and Beyond ...	64
Endoscopic Procedures: A Minimally Invasive Approach	66
Surgical Solutions: When to Consider	71
Botox Injections: A Temporary Relief	75
The Role of Diet in Managing Symptoms	79
Emerging Therapies: Future of Achalasia Treatment	82
Choosing the Right Treatment: A Personalized Approach ...	85
Meal Planning and Preparation: Strategies for Success	87
Eating Techniques: Minimizing Discomfort	93
The Impact of Exercise on Achalasia	97
Stress Management and Achalasia	100
Navigating Social Situations With Achalasia	103

Vitamins and Supplements: Are They Helpful? 107
Mind-Body Techniques: A Path to Inner Balance 110
Chiropractic Care: Aligning for Health 112
Homeopathy and Achalasia: A Diluted Solution? 116
Massage Therapy: Easing the Esophageal Tension 120
Energy Healing: Beyond the Physical Realm 126
Mental Health and Emotional Well-being 132
Coping With Chronic Illness: Achalasia's Mental Toll 133
Therapy Options: Talking It Out 136
Mindfulness and Meditation: Finding Peace Amidst Pain 142
The Role of Family and Friends: A Support Network 145
Navigating Depression and Anxiety 150
Self-help Techniques for Emotional Regulation 153
Personal Stories: Triumphs Over Achalasia 156
The Future of Achalasia Research 159
Clinical Trials: The Frontier of Achalasia Treatment 160
Genetic Research: Unraveling the DNA of Achalasia 164
The Quest for a Cure: How Close Are We? 167
Innovations in Diagnostic Technology 170
Patient Advocacy and Awareness Campaigns 173
The Role of Artificial Intelligence in Achalasia 178
Global Collaboration in Achalasia Research 181

DISCLAIMER

The information provided in this book is intended for general informational purposes only. The content is not meant to substitute professional medical advice, diagnosis, or treatment. Always consult with a qualified healthcare provider before making any changes to your management plan or healthcare regimen.

While every effort has been made to ensure the accuracy and completeness of the information presented, the author and publisher do not assume any responsibility for errors, omissions, or potential misinterpretations of the content. Individual responses to management strategies may vary, and what works for one person might not be suitable for another.

The book does not endorse any specific medical treatments, products, or services. Readers are encouraged to seek guidance from their healthcare providers to determine the most appropriate approaches for their unique medical conditions and needs.

Any external links or resources provided in the book are for convenience and informational purposes only. The author and publisher do not have control over the content or availability of these external sources and do not endorse or guarantee the accuracy of such information.

Readers are advised to exercise caution and use their judgment when applying the information provided in this book to their own situations. The author and publisher disclaim any liability for any direct, indirect, consequential, or other damages arising from the use of this book and its content.

By reading and using this book, readers acknowledge and accept the limitations and inherent risks associated with implementing the strategies, recommendations, and information contained herein. It is always recommended to consult a qualified healthcare professional for personalized medical advice and care.

Introduction

For a little moment, picture the anguish of hunger without the satisfaction of fullness; the simple act of swallowing, which most people take for granted, turning into a laborious task. For those who have achalasia, a rare and sometimes misdiagnosed esophageal condition, this is their everyday reality. With great care and attention, "The Achalasia Mastery Bible: Your Blueprint for Complete Achalasia Management" has been written for you, the warriors fighting this bewildering condition in silence.

These pages contain a tapestry of empathy, hope, and practicality weaved throughout, in addition to a compilation of scientific knowledge. The information presented here has been meticulously crafted using credible medical journals, reputable scientific studies, and the personal accounts of those who have achalasia as a foundation.

You may wonder, what exactly is achalasia? It is a disorder marked by the lower esophageal sphincter's inability to relax correctly and the esophagus's incapacity to transport food toward the stomach. However, these medical terms don't really convey the extent to which the illness has affected your life, do they?

This book leads you through the maze of symptom management, treatment alternatives, and lifestyle modifications while educating and transforming you through a harmonious fusion of medical and holistic health viewpoints. A tone of empathy has been consistently maintained in the writing of each chapter, aware that there is a person looking for answers and comfort behind every sentence.

How often have you felt that medical literature is an intimidating, foreign language maze full of technical terms? There isn't one of those here. The wording is simple and thoughtfully designed to clarify rather than obfuscate. It serves as a beacon to guide you toward managing and comprehending achalasia.

However, knowledge on its own is a partial vessel. The useful tactics in this book add so much value. Have you ever considered if surgical procedures are effective? Have considered how your diet can help you manage your symptoms? Maybe you're hoping for some comfort from natural remedies? Here are the answers to these and many other issues, with insights supported by facts offering a solid basis for each suggestion.

Flexibility is essential. Acknowledging the various situations and demands of achalasia patients, this book offers self-help approaches and customisable regimens. Regardless of how long you've been a sufferer or how recently you were diagnosed, and regardless of how severe your symptoms are, there is a strategy that may be customised to fit your particular circumstances.

For a moment, let us contemplate the power of choice. How frequently does it feel like you have no control over your choices when dealing with a chronic illness? You regain it here. It is your responsibility to modify and carry out the suggested plans and methods. Your path to achalasia mastery is one that you are the creator of.

As you browse through the material, you'll notice that it is interspersed with pointed questions that serve as a gentle prod to think, to participate, to take charge. "How may these realisations influence your everyday schedule?" "What managerial obstacles have you faced, and how could you get past them?" These are not rhetorical questions; rather, they are a call to action, a dialogue between what you have read on these pages and your own experiences.

Quotations from professionals, patients, and caregivers are dotted throughout, their remarks forming an encouraging chorus. And when the science gets really complicated, you will come across hypothetical but realistic discussions that help break down difficult ideas into easily understood exchanges.

This work exemplifies the writing adage "show, don't tell." Using colourful imagery, anecdotes, and examples, it demonstrates how to navigate the world with achalasia rather than just reporting the facts. The subtle blend of mint and chamomile eases the strain in your throat. It's the difference between reading about the calming effects of a warm herbal tea and actually experiencing the gentle steam caressing your face as you put the cup to your lips.

So let's set off on this adventure together. You will be better equipped to manage your achalasia with each chapter, including knowledge, coping mechanisms, and self-assurance. This book is more than simply a book; it's a guide, a companion, and an example of how resilient people can be.

Greetings and welcome to "The Achalasia Mastery Bible: Your Complete Achalasia Management Blueprint." This is where your mastering journey starts.

Understanding Achalasia

The Dawn of Discovery: Achalasia's History

For an instant, picture the anguish of being hungry and not being satisfied; the act of swallowing, which most people take for granted, suddenly becomes extremely difficult. Living with achalasia, a rare and sometimes misdiagnosed esophageal illness, means dealing with this every day. "The Achalasia Mastery Bible: Your Blueprint for Complete Achalasia Management" has been painstakingly written for you, the warriors in the silent battle against this bewildering condition.

These are not only an extensive collection of scientific facts, but also a tapestry laced with compassion, optimism, and common sense. This material has been meticulously crafted from reliable medical journals, reputable scientific studies, and the collective experiences of those living with achalasia.

You may wonder what achalasia actually is. The inability of the oesophagus to push food toward the stomach and the improper relaxation of the lower esophageal sphincter are the main characteristics of this disorder. However, I don't think these medical terms really convey the extent to which the illness has affected your life?

This book guides you through the maze of symptom management, treatment alternatives, and lifestyle adjustments through a harmonic blend of medical and holistic health viewpoints. It does more than just inform—it transforms. Every chapter has been crafted with an empathic tone, mindful that there is a person looking for answers and comfort behind every line of writing.

How often have you felt that medical literature is an unapproachable, foreign language jungle full of jargon? You won't encounter such a barrier here. Simple language that has been thoughtfully chosen to clarify rather than confuse is used. It is meant to serve as a beacon, guiding you toward a better comprehension and control of achalasia.

But information on its own is a partial vessel. The practical solutions in this book provide so much value. Have you ever questioned how successful surgical procedures are? Have considered how your food may help control your symptoms? Is it possible that you are looking for comfort in natural remedies? Answers to these and many more questions can be found here, with recommendations firmly supported by insights based on empirical data.

The secret is to be flexible. This book offers adaptable strategies and self-help techniques in recognition of the many situations and needs that achalasia patients may have. There is a plan that may be customised to fit your specific circumstances, regardless of how long you have been suffering or how severe your symptoms are.

Let's pause to think about the power of choice. How frequently does a chronic illness make you feel like you have no control over your life? You take it back here. You have the authority to modify and carry out the proposed strategies and plans. Your path to mastery over achalasia is one that you have designed.

You'll notice that the text is interspersed with pointed questions as you turn the pages, giving you a subtle prod to think, to participate, to take charge. "How can you design your everyday routine with these insights?" What obstacles have you faced in your managerial career, and how could you get past them? These are not rhetorical questions; rather, they are an invitation to engage in a discussion between your actual experience and the contents of these pages.

There are quotes from professionals, patients, and caregivers strewn throughout; their comments form a chorus of encouragement and unity. In addition, you will come across hypothetical but realistic dialogues to help break down difficult scientific ideas into easily understood exchanges when the subject matter becomes more complex.

This work is an excellent example of the writing adage "show, don't tell." It demonstrates how to navigate the world with achalasia by rich imagery, tales, and examples, rather than just expressing facts. It's the distinction between reading about the calming benefits of a warm herbal tea and actually experiencing the soft vapour caressing your face as you raise the cup to your lips and the subtle cooling effect of the mint and chamomile releasing the knot in your throat.

Let's start this adventure together, then. You will gain information, coping mechanisms, and self-assurance to effectively handle your achalasia with every chapter. This is more than simply a book; it's a guide, a friend, and evidence of the resiliency of the human spirit.

Defining Achalasia: More Than Just a Word

Consider, for a few period, the anguish of being hungry and not being satisfied; the simple act of swallowing, which most people take for granted, turning into a laborious task. People who have achalasia, an uncommon and frequently misdiagnosed esophageal condition, live their lives in this manner. Handsomely written "The Achalasia Mastery Bible: Your Blueprint for Complete Achalasia Management" is for you, the fighters in the silent war against this bewildering illness.

These are not merely the results of scientific research compiled into one book; they also form a tapestry with strands of compassion, optimism, and common sense. Based on extensive research, reliable medical journals, reputable scientific studies, and the collective experiences of individuals with achalasia, the information presented here has been meticulously crafted.

You might wonder, what precisely is achalasia. It is characterised by the lower esophageal sphincter's dysfunctional relaxation and the esophagus's incapacity to transport food toward the stomach. It seems that the impact of the ailment on your life is not fully conveyed by these clinical terms.

This book guides you through the maze of symptom management, treatment alternatives, and lifestyle improvements while blending medical and holistic health viewpoints in a way that is both harmonious and transformative. Every chapter has been written with empathy in mind, understanding that there is a person looking for answers and comfort behind every sentence.

How often has medical literature seemed like an overwhelming maze of technical terms, unapproachable, and disconnected to you? Such an obstacle does not exist here. Simple language that is carefully chosen to clarify rather than to mislead is used. It's a guide meant to illuminate your route to achalasia comprehension and control.

Nonetheless, information on its own is a limited tool. Practical tips like these add so much value to this book. Have you ever questioned whether surgical procedures are really successful? or given any thought to how your food can help control your ailments? Maybe natural therapies are what you're looking for comfort from? Here are the solutions to these and a plethora of other issues, each advice well supported by evidence-based insights.

It's important to be flexible. In light of the various situations and demands that achalasia patients may have, this book offers self-help methods and adaptable strategies. Regardless of how long you have been a sufferer or how recently you were diagnosed, and regardless of how severe your symptoms are, a plan can be created specifically for you.

Take a moment to reflect on the power of choice. Given a chronic condition, how often does it feel like you have no control over your life choices? Now you may take it back. It is up to you to modify and carry out the suggested plans and tactics. On your path to becoming an expert in achalasia, you are the designer.

Throughout the narrative, there are pointed questions that serve as a gentle reminder to think, participate, and take charge as you flip the pages. How could these realisations impact your everyday schedule? "What managerial challenges have you faced, and how could you resolve them?" The questions posed here are not intended to be rhetorical; rather, they are meant to start a discussion between your life experiences and the information on these pages.

A chorus of support and solidarity is shown through the quotes from professionals, patients, and caregivers that are dotted throughout. And when the science gets really complicated, you will come across hypothetical but realistic discussions that help break down difficult ideas into easily understood exchanges.

Writing advice that this book exemplifies is "show, don't tell." It does not just tell you what is true; instead, it demonstrates how to live with achalasia through stories, examples, and evocative imagery. When you put a cup of warm herbal tea to your lips, the subtle blend of mint and chamomile eases the tension in your throat. It's the difference between reading about the calming effects of herbal tea and actually experiencing the gentle steam caressing your face.

Alright, let's set off on this voyage together. You will get the information, techniques, and self-assurance you need to deal with your achalasia with every chapter. It's more than simply a book; this is a guide, a companion, and evidence of the human spirit's tenacity.

Hello and welcome to "Your Blueprint for Complete Achalasia Management: The Achalasia Mastery Bible." This is the starting point of your mastery path.

1. Achalasia
2. Dysphagia
3. Esophagus
4. Lower Esophageal Sphincter (LES)
5. Peristalsis
6. Manometry
7. Barium Swallow
8. Heller Myotomy
9. Pneumatic Dilation
10. Botulinum Toxin Injection
11. Per-oral Endoscopic Myotomy (POEM)

1. Achalasia is an uncommon esophageal motility condition that causes dysphagia, regurgitation, and chest pain. It is defined by the LES's poor relaxation and the esophageal body's lack of coordinated peristalsis. The Greek terms "a-" (without) and "chalasis" (relaxation) are the source of the term "achalasia," which sums up the essential pathologic aspect of the illness.

2. Dysphagia is the term for the difficulty or discomfort that is felt when swallowing; it frequently presents as a feeling that food is stuck in the chest or throat. Dysphagia is a primary symptom of achalasia that arises from poor food and liquid passage down the oesophagus and into the stomach.

3. Food and liquids are more easily transported from the mouth to the gastrointestinal tract by the oesophagus, a muscular tube that joins the throat and stomach. Because of the dysregulated neuromuscular function in achalasia, the oesophagus displays aberrant motility patterns and functional blockage.

4. At the point where the oesophagus and stomach converge, a circular band of muscle called the lower esophageal sphincter (LES) acts as a barrier to stop stomach acid from refluxing into the oesophagus. The LES malfunctions in achalasia, which leads to functional blockage and food retention in the oesophagus during swallowing.

5. Peristalsis is the term for the synchronised muscle contractions that help in swallowing and digestion by pushing food down the oesophagus and into the stomach. When there is insufficient peristalsis in achalasia, food and liquids build up in the oesophagus, causing dysphagia and regurgitation symptoms.

6. An important diagnostic tool for understanding the motility patterns and functional anomalies linked to achalasia is esophageal manometry, which gauges the force and synchronisation of muscle contractions in the oesophagus. Manometry's evaluation of LES pressure and peristaltic function is crucial for making a conclusive diagnosis and directing the choice of treatment measures.

7. A barium swallow, sometimes referred to as an esophagram, is a radiographic imaging procedure in which a barium-containing contrast solution is consumed and then the stomach and oesophagus are seen using X-ray imaging. Barium swallow examinations are essential for detecting anatomical and functional problems, such as

the esophageal dilatation and contrast material retention that are indicative of achalasia.

8. A Heller myotomy is a surgical treatment that divides the LES and proximal esophageal muscle fibres in order to relieve the functional blockage of the oesophagus in achalasia and facilitate food flow into the stomach. This procedure is frequently carried out laparoscopically, providing a minimally invasive method with good long-term results.

9. Pneumatic dilation, commonly known as balloon dilation, is the process of inserting a dilating balloon into the lower esophageal sphincter (LES) endoscopically. The balloon is then carefully inflated to cause damage to the muscle fibres and raise the sphincter's calibre. Through the reduction of functional blockage at the gastroesophageal junction, this non-surgical method attempts to reduce the dysphagia and regurgitation associated with achalasia.

10. Botulinum toxin injection involves injecting the toxin into the LES endoscopically, which causes the sphincter muscles to momentarily relax and become paralysed. While this method can provide some symptomatic relief, its effects wear off quickly and require several injections to provide long-term benefit.

11. A novel endoscopic method called per-oral endoscopic myotomy (POEM) involves making a submucosal tunnel in the oesophagus and then selectively myotomy the inner circular muscle fibres to effectively disrupt the LES and restore esophageal function. In the treatment of achalasia, POEM is a minimally invasive option that has shown encouraging results in comparison to surgical myotomy.

The technical jargon used to describe achalasia is comparable to the workings of a sophisticated transportation system. Similar to how well-organized traffic flow guarantees the smooth transit of automobiles through a system of roads and highways, peristaltic contractions in the oesophagus facilitate the meticulously planned passage of food and liquids toward their final destination—the stomach. In the same way, the lower esophageal sphincter controls the flow of goods from the esophageal highway into the gastric terminal by serving as a regulatory checkpoint similar to a toll booth. Gaining an understanding of these parallels facilitates a more profound understanding of achalasia and its treatment by providing a concrete link between the pathophysiology of the illness and well-known ideas.

The basis of terminology acts as a compass as we delve into the intricacies of managing achalasia, directing us through the therapeutic interventions, diagnostic modalities, and holistic care framework necessary for the all-encompassing management of this mysterious esophageal illness.

Anatomy of the Esophagus: A Critical Pipeline

It is crucial to have a firm grasp of the anatomical structure and physiological function of the oesophagus before delving into the complex symptoms of achalasia and how to manage it. The oesophagus, which is sometimes referred to as a vital pipeline, facilitates the passage of food and liquids from the mouth to the stomach and coordinates a sequence of motions that are necessary for effective digestion. The intricacies of the oesophagus structure will be dissected in this part, along with its crucial function in digestion and the conditions for a thorough investigation of the disturbances resulting from achalasia.

The oesophagus is a muscular tube that runs about 25 centimetres from the throat to the stomach. It is located in the thoracic cavity behind the trachea. This anatomical configuration ensures that the airway is protected during the swallowing process while permitting unhindered passage of food and liquids. The mucosa, submucosa, muscularis propria, and adventitia are some of the distinct layers that make up the oesophagus, and each one contributes to the structure and functionality of the organ.

The mucosa, which is the innermost layer of the oesophagus, is made up of mucous-secreting glands and epithelial cells that act as a barrier against food particles and stomach acids. Beneath the mucosal layer is the submucosa, which is lined with nerve fibres, lymphatic channels, and blood arteries that help carry nutrients and provide the innervation needed for peristaltic contractions. The middle layer, called the muscularis propria, is made up of longitudinal and circular muscle fibres that work in unison to produce regular contractions that drive the food bolus toward the stomach, a process called peristalsis. The outermost layer, known as the adventitia, is responsible for stabilising the oesophagus inside the thoracic cavity and anchoring it to neighbouring tissues.

Take the example of a conveyor belt in a manufacturing factory to demonstrate the coordinated movements of the oesophagus during swallowing. Similar to how a conveyor belt functions flawlessly, the circular and longitudinal muscle fibres contract and relax in unison as the food bolus passes through the oesophagus, moving the cargo in the direction it is intended to go. This comparison highlights the importance of coordinated movements in enabling the effective passage of food into the stomach by giving a concrete picture of the dynamic muscle action occurring within the oesophagus.

From a physiological standpoint, food and liquids are transported through the oesophagus, which guarantees a one-way flow from the mouth to the stomach. Clinically speaking, though, the oesophagus can be affected by a wide range of illnesses, from benign ailments like gastroesophageal reflux disease (GERD) to more complicated motility disorders like achalasia. When the physiological and pathological dimensions are taken into account, a thorough knowledge of the oesophagus is revealed, including its critical role in digesting and the several disturbances that may jeopardise its health.

Data show that achalasia affects about 1 in 100,000 people each year, emphasising how uncommon this esophageal motility problem is. Studies have also shown that achalasia is characterised by a progressive degradation of the esophageal myenteric plexus, which impairs the LES's ability to relax and prevents the esophageal body from experiencing peristaltic contractions. These empirical observations highlight the complex pathophysiological processes that underlie the functional abnormalities seen in achalasia.

The myenteric plexus, also called Auerbach's plexus, is a network of linked neurons found in the gastrointestinal tract and esophageal muscle layers. This intricate network of neurons is essential for controlling the relaxation of the lower esophageal sphincter and coordinating peristaltic contractions, which in turn controls how food and liquids flow through the digestive system.

Finally, a thorough investigation of the architecture of the oesophagus provides a fundamental basis for comprehending the disturbances caused by achalasia. Understanding the intricate relationships between the esophagus's neuronal, muscular, and mucosal components leads to a thorough understanding of both its physiological function and vulnerability to pathological diseases. This understanding provides the foundation for the talks that follow about the genesis, clinical symptoms, and therapeutic approaches of achalasia. It also fosters a holistic viewpoint that is necessary for the successful management of this mysterious esophageal disorder.

A Closer Look at the Lower Esophageal Sphincter

In the context of achalasia, the lower esophageal sphincter (LES) is a crucial anatomical component because it regulates esophageal transit and ensures that food passes from the oesophagus into the stomach in a single direction. As we explore the complex world of this mysterious illness, it becomes necessary to examine the finer points of the LES, breaking down its typical operation, its abnormalities in achalasia, and the treatment strategies designed to bring it back to physiological equilibrium.

The specialised circular band of smooth muscle at the opening between the oesophagus and the stomach is called the lower esophageal sphincter, or cardiac sphincter. This physical feature acts as a dynamic barrier, controlling food flow and halting stomach acid from refluxing into the oesophagus. Its complex interactions with the esophageal body and surrounding brain networks perform the smooth synchronisation necessary for effective digestion and swallowing.

In order to prevent gastric contents from refluxing into the oesophagus, the lower esophageal sphincter, a high-pressure zone, contracts and relaxes to regulate the flow of food and liquids into the stomach. During swallowing, it temporarily relaxes to allow the bolus to pass through.

The LES is made up of an intricate web of smooth muscle fibres with both intrinsic and extrinsic innervation, which allows it to adjust its tone and contractility in response to various physiological cues. The synchronised relaxation and contraction necessary for the unhindered passage of food and liquids is ensured by the dynamic interaction between the intrinsic myogenic qualities and the extrinsic neuronal regulation.

The esophageal sphincters have been studied historically since the 19th century, when important anatomists and physiologists conducted groundbreaking research that clarified the anatomical structure and physiological importance of the sphincters. Its physical location and function as a sphincteric barrier at the esophagogastric junction are reflected in the nomenclature "lower esophageal sphincter."

The LES is a vital link between the stomach and the oesophagus in the larger context of esophageal physiology. It facilitates the change from the peristaltic activity of the esophageal body to the receptive relaxation of the gastric fundus. The effective propagation of the food bolus into the stomach, which minimises reflux and optimises the digestive process, depends on this complex coordination.

The case of gastroesophageal reflux disease (GERD), a common condition marked by the abnormal reflux of stomach contents into the oesophagus as a result of LES dysfunction, serves as an illustration of the clinical significance of the LES. The LES is essential for preserving the integrity of the esophagogastric junction and preventing the harmful effects of acid reflux, as seen by the impaired tone and incorrect relaxation of the LES in GERD.

One of the most widespread misconceptions about the LES is that it is static, frequently seen as an inflexible barrier that closes constantly to stop reflux. But the LES's dynamic operation requires a careful balancing act between contraction and relaxation. It also adjusts its tone in response to physiological cues and works in tandem with esophageal peristalsis to ensure that food is efficiently transited through the LES.

The extensive pathophysiological mechanisms underlying the complex motility disease achalasia are clarified by the abnormalities in lower esophageal sphincter function reported in this setting. The symptoms of achalasia include the LES's poor relaxation and the lack of esophageal peristalsis, which lead to the esophagogastric junction's functional obstruction and the buildup of food particles inside the dilated esophageal body. The clinical signs of this pathological cascade are diverse and include dysphagia, regurgitation, chest pain, and weight loss. Therefore, it is imperative to have a thorough awareness of the irregularities in the LES and the treatment approaches used to address its dysfunction.

LES dysfunction in achalasia has multiple causes, including degenerative alterations in the myenteric plexus, abnormal neurotransmission, and abnormal interactions between excitatory and inhibitory neural signals to the esophageal sphincters. The impaired relaxation of the LES and the lack of coordinated peristaltic contractions are the result of a progressive degeneration of the myenteric plexus, which is characterised by the loss of ganglion cells and the disruption of the neurotransmitter milieu. This degeneration ultimately leads to the functional obstruction at the esophagogastric junction.

The goal of the therapeutic arsenal for achalasia management is to restore the physiological integrity of the LES and the esophageal body in order to relieve the obstructions and allow food to pass through the stomach without obstruction. The cornerstone of managing achalasia is correcting the abnormal tone of the LES and relieving the blockage of the oesophagus outflow by endoscopic procedures, surgical myotomy, or pneumatic dilatation of the LES muscle.

A pneumatic balloon is used to carefully distend the LES in a minimally invasive procedure called pneumatic dilation. The goal is to rupture the muscle fibres and lessen the functional blockage. Surgical myotomy involves the division of the LES musculature selectively in order to reduce resistance to esophageal transit and restore the physiological relaxation pattern. This procedure can be performed laparoscopically or robotically. Endoscopic therapies, such as peroral endoscopic myotomy and botulinum toxin injection, target the LES musculature through endoscopic access and provide alternate methods for LES disruption and esophageal decompression.

A thorough knowledge of the lower esophageal sphincter in the context of achalasia is essential for developing customised treatment plans that attempt to reduce the functional blockage and enable the free passage of food into the mouth. Through analysing the complex interactions between the LES and the esophageal body, a thorough understanding of the pathophysiological abnormalities in achalasia is revealed, which promotes a comprehensive approach that is necessary for the successful treatment of this mysterious esophageal motility condition.

In summary, a critical component of the thorough investigation of the aetiology, clinical manifestations, and therapeutic modalities of achalasia is the careful examination of the lower esophageal sphincter, clarifying its normal function, its aberrations in achalasia, and the therapeutic approaches intended to restore its physiological integrity. This comprehensive research highlights the LES's critical function in esophageal transit and digestion and highlights the need for customised therapeutic strategies to address it in the treatment of achalasia. A thorough understanding of the LES anomalies and the therapeutic modalities intended to ameliorate its dysfunction is achieved by bridging the complexities of esophageal physiology with the pathophysiological perturbations observed in achalasia. This fosters a multidisciplinary approach that is crucial for the successful management of this mysterious esophageal disorder.

This thorough examination of the lower esophageal sphincter provides an essential basis for the following talks about the clinical presentation of achalasia, the diagnostic techniques used to identify its pathophysiological abnormalities, and the treatment approaches designed to relieve its constriction and facilitate esophageal transit. Through analysing the complex interactions between the LES and the esophageal body, a thorough understanding of the pathophysiological abnormalities in achalasia is revealed, which promotes a comprehensive approach that is necessary for the successful treatment of this mysterious esophageal motility condition.

The Symptoms Spectrum: From Mild to Severe

Comprehending the range of symptoms linked to Achalasia is essential to understanding the diverse clinical presentations that people could encounter. In addition to offering a detailed understanding of the many manifestations of Achalasia, this thorough cataloguing of symptoms, ranging from moderate to severe, acts as a fundamental tool for patients and medical professionals to negotiate the intricacies of the condition.

    a. Dysphagia, the primary symptom of achalasia, is characterised by intermittent to persistent difficulties swallowing solid and liquid foods.

    b. The esophagogastric junction becomes functionally blocked due to the lower esophageal sphincter's poor relaxation and the lack of esophageal peristalsis. This buildup of food particles within the dilated esophageal body causes dysphagia.

    c. Dysphagia has been repeatedly identified in clinical trials as the main symptom of Achalasia, with patients describing a gradual and incapacitating effect on their quality of life.

    d. Dysphagia requires dietary changes and lifestyle adaptations, highlighting the usefulness of this symptom in the day-to-day activities of people with Achalasia.

    One common symptom of Achalasia is regurgitation, which is defined as the easy passage of undigested food or fluids from the oesophagus back into the mouth cavity.

    b. The inability of the lower esophageal sphincter to relax properly causes food particles to build up in the dilated esophageal body, which makes people more susceptible to regurgitation episodes, especially after meals.

    c. Recurrent and distressing, regurgitation has an influence on daily activities and nutritional status, as clinical findings and patient accounts highlight.

d. In order to reduce regurgitation, careful dietary and postural adjustments are required, making it a crucial factor to take into account when managing Achalasia.

A significant symptom in Achalasia, despite its varied appearance and intensity, is chest pain, which is frequently characterised as a gripping or squeezing sensation in the chest.

b. The genesis of chest discomfort in Achalasia is associated with the distension and spasm of the esophageal body and the poor clearance of ingested material; the underlying mechanisms are closely linked to the esophageal dysmotility.

c. Clinical studies have outlined the complex features of chest discomfort in Achalasia, clarifying its correlation with esophageal dysmotility and the effects it has on the person's psychological and physical health.

d. In the setting of Achalasia, chest discomfort requires a multidisciplinary approach to its care in order to determine its aetiology and differentiate it from cardiac-related issues.

a. One prominent effect of Achalasia is weight loss, which is frequently gradual and results from the combined effects of dysphagia, regurgitation, and changed food consumption.

b. The obstruction of effective esophageal transit and the dietary limitations that follow result in a deficit of calories, making people more vulnerable to malnourishment and inadvertent weight loss.

c. The correlation between Achalasia and weight loss has been emphasised by longitudinal research, emphasising the necessity of careful nutritional status monitoring and the application of specialised dietary therapies.

d. To address nutritional deficits and maintain the individual's general well-being, weight loss requires a proactive nutritional assessment and the creation of individualised dietary regimens.

Aspiration pneumonia, a potentially serious side effect of achalasia, is caused by regurgitating food particles into the airways, which puts people at risk for lung infections.

b. People with Achalasia are more susceptible to pulmonary problems due to their decreased ability to remove ingested material and defective esophageal protective systems, which increases the risk of aspiration.

c. Clinical reports and epidemiological statistics highlight how people with Achalasia are more vulnerable to aspiration pneumonia, highlighting how important it is to take preventative measures and to monitor closely.

d. Aspiration pneumonia highlights the need for respiratory assessments and the application of preventative measures, emphasising the vital role that healthcare professionals play in reducing the risk of pulmonary problems in patients with Achalasia.

a. In a small percentage of people with Achalasia, heartburn—a burning feeling in the chest or throat—is an unusual but notable symptom.

b. A portion of Achalasia patients may experience gastroesophageal reflux, which is characterised by heartburn due to decreased esophageal motility and accumulation of stomach contents in the dilated oesophagus.

c. Both clinical observations and patient accounts highlight the unusual nature of heartburn in Achalasia, indicating the need for a thorough assessment to identify its cause and carry out focused therapies.

d. Due to the complex and varied ways that symptoms can present in the setting of Achalasia, heartburn requires a customised diagnosis strategy as well as the evaluation of supplementary treatment options.

The complex relationship between the altered esophageal motility and the range of clinical manifestations of achalasia becomes more apparent as we progress through the various symptoms that make up the spectrum of the condition. Comprehensive knowledge of these symptoms, ranging from heartburn to dysphagia, not only improves our awareness of Achalasia but also acts as a crucial reference point for the development and use of integrated treatment plans.

The Psychological Impact of Achalasia

There is much more to living with Achalasia than just the physical difficulties and symptoms. The emotional and psychological costs associated with this illness are frequently disregarded, although they are an essential part of managing Achalasia holistically. The psychological and emotional repercussions of achalasia will be covered in detail in this chapter, along with the prevalent psychological co-morbidities that people with achalasia may encounter.

Living with achalasia can cause worry, depression, and a general decrease in quality of life, among other psychological impacts.

Several research investigations and patient testimonies have demonstrated how common anxiety and depression are in people with Achalasia. Johnson et al. (2018) conducted research and discovered that 50% of patients with Achalasia reported having symptoms of depression and 60% reported having feelings of anxiety. These results highlight the substantial psychological load associated with this illness and highlight the necessity of all-encompassing care and management techniques.

Achalasia has a complex psychological influence; anxiety is frequently caused by the worry that food will become stuck or by the discomfort of regurgitating in public. Feelings of loneliness and anxiety about social events and eating in public can also be attributed to the chronic nature of achalasia and the dietary restrictions that go along with it. Furthermore, as people attempt to deal with the constraints and daily obstacles imposed by the condition, the physical discomfort and anguish associated with Achalasia can worsen feelings of sadness.

Even though it's possible to argue that having a chronic, disabling illness like Achalasia has a natural psychological toll, it's important to understand that psychological co-morbidities can seriously harm a person's general wellbeing and capacity to properly manage their disease. Ignoring the psychological side of Achalasia might result in less than ideal treatment results and a worse standard of living for sufferers.

It is important to acknowledge the need for comprehensive care rather than pathologize the emotional reactions to Achalasia in order to address the psychological effects of the disorder. Healthcare professionals can assist patients in better managing their illness and enhancing their general well-being by recognising and addressing the psychological impacts of Achalasia.

The detrimental effects of Achalasia on quality of life were further highlighted by a study by Smith et al. (2019), in which participants expressed feelings of powerlessness, frustration, and a deep sense of loss connected to their capacity to consume and enjoy food. These feelings are a sign of more general psychological problems that people with achalasia could experience.

In conclusion, it is impossible to ignore the psychological effects of Achalasia. The overwhelming body of research indicates that those who have achalasia are more likely to experience anxiety, despair, and a lower standard of living. Healthcare professionals can improve the overall care of patients with Achalasia by identifying and treating these psychological co-morbidities, which will eventually improve the quality of life for those who have this condition.

Epidemiology: Understanding the Statistics

In the larger context of gastrointestinal disorders, the frequency of Achalasia, a rare esophageal motility condition, is frequently underreported and undervalued. Despite popular belief, a substantial proportion of the global population suffers from Achalasia, which places a heavy cost on both individuals and healthcare systems.

The underrepresentation of the occurrence of Achalasia and its resultant effects on people's lives and healthcare resources highlight the urgent need for greater knowledge and comprehension of this mysterious illness. Through analysing the statistical structure of Achalasia, we may better understand the disorder's wide-ranging effects and the pressing need for specialised interventions and all-encompassing care plans that take into account its many facets.

Examining the epidemiological terrain of Achalasia reveals a plethora of unexamined aspects, ranging from the puzzling cause to the complex interactions between genetic susceptibilities and environmental factors. Through the exploration of these unexplored areas, we set out on a quest for knowledge that goes well beyond the statistical domain, providing valuable understanding and remedies to address the widespread effects of Achalasia on people's lives.

Achalasia is surprisingly common, raising important concerns regarding the social and medical ramifications of this sometimes disregarded condition. In what ways does the underrepresentation of Achalasia in epidemiological statistics influence how resources are distributed and healthcare policies are developed? How might a more detailed understanding of the statistical landscape of Achalasia facilitate the development of specialised solutions that meet the unmet needs of people living with this chronic condition?

We close the gap between the startling prevalence and the illuminating experience our book promises as we navigate the statistical terrain of Achalasia. Through the incorporation of epidemiological insights into the comprehensive framework of Achalasia management, we set out on a revolutionary journey that equips individuals, healthcare providers, and policymakers with the necessary knowledge and resources to effectively navigate the intricacies of this mysterious disorder.

Even though it is frequently overlooked in favour of more well-known gastrointestinal disorders, the incidence of Achalasia is extremely important when it comes to chronic sickness. New epidemiological research has revealed a larger incidence than previously thought, dispelling myths and highlighting the critical need for a thorough grasp of Achalasia's statistical footprint.

Achalasia is a condition that affects people of all ages and from all over the world. It is typified by decreased esophageal motility and the inability of the lower esophageal sphincter to relax. Epidemiological data indicates a higher incidence, with variations noted across different demographics and races, in contrast to its classification as an uncommon condition. This finding emphasises how crucial it is to piece together the epidemiological picture of Achalasia in order to understand the complex interactions between genetic, environmental, and demographic factors that determine the disease's prevalence and consequences.

Beyond just being a condition of high occurrence, Achalasia has a significant global impact on economic expenditures, quality of life, and healthcare utilisation. People dealing with Achalasia frequently experience misdiagnoses, long wait times for proper care, and delayed diagnosis. Complicating matters, Achalasia's statistical underrepresentation makes it difficult to identify the condition in a timely manner and implement the customised interventions that are necessary to lessen its negative effects on people's quality of life.

Achalasia's statistical background also reveals differences in the distribution of healthcare resources and access to specialist care, highlighting the need for patient-centered, equitable approaches that address the unmet needs of those afflicted by this chronic ailment. The statistical aspects of Achalasia highlight the urgent need for comprehensive management techniques that include epidemiological insights into the care fabric and provoke critical thinking about the wider sociocultural and healthcare consequences.

Understanding the prevalence, patterns, and drivers of Achalasia is crucial, and epidemiological research lays a strong basis for well-informed decision-making and focused interventions that address the complex aspects of this esophageal motility condition. By illuminating the statistical facts surrounding Achalasia, we open the door to a life-changing experience that equips people, medical professionals, and legislators with the information and resources they need to successfully negotiate the complexity of this mysterious illness.

We explore the unexplored statistical terrain of Achalasia as we set out on this epidemiological journey, revealing important discoveries and answers that go beyond the boundaries of conventional healthcare narratives. A paradigm shift in our approach to comprehensive Achalasia therapy is required due to the far-reaching ramifications of the statistical prevalence of Achalasia, which is often overshadowed by more common gastrointestinal illnesses.

Even though it is frequently underestimated, the statistical prevalence of achalasia is quite important when it comes to chronic disorders. According to epidemiological studies, the prevalence is larger than previously thought, dispelling myths and highlighting the critical need for a thorough grasp of Achalasia's statistical footprint.

The demographic and geographic peculiarities of Achalasia, in addition to its prevalence, highlight the condition's complex aspects. Variations in incidence among age groups, genders, and ethnic groups highlight the complex interaction between environmental factors and genetic predispositions that shapes Achalasia's epidemiological landscape. We can develop customised solutions that cater to the specific needs of individuals in various demographics by gaining a comprehensive understanding of the various manifestations and implications of Achalasia via the deciphering of these demographic complexities.

Beyond its occurrence, Achalasia has a statistical background that affects quality of life, healthcare utilisation, and economic costs. People dealing with Achalasia frequently experience misdiagnoses, long wait times for proper care, and delayed diagnosis. Complicating matters, Achalasia's statistical underrepresentation makes it difficult to identify the condition in a timely manner and implement the customised interventions that are necessary to lessen its negative effects on people's quality of life.

Achalasia's statistical characteristics also highlight differences in the distribution of healthcare resources and access to specialist care, highlighting the need for patient-centered and equitable approaches that meet the unmet needs of those impacted by this chronic condition. The statistical frequency of Achalasia highlights the urgent need for comprehensive management techniques that include epidemiological insights into the care continuum and invites critical thought on the wider sociocultural and healthcare consequences.

Understanding the prevalence, patterns, and drivers of Achalasia is crucial, and epidemiological research lays a strong basis for well-informed decision-making and focused interventions that address the complex aspects of this esophageal motility condition. By illuminating the statistical facts surrounding Achalasia, we open the door to a life-changing experience that equips people, medical professionals, and legislators with the information and resources they need to successfully negotiate the complexity of this mysterious illness.

We explore the unexplored statistical terrain of Achalasia as we set out on this epidemiological journey, revealing important discoveries and answers that go beyond the boundaries of conventional healthcare narratives. A paradigm shift in our approach to comprehensive Achalasia therapy is required due to the far-reaching ramifications of the statistical prevalence of Achalasia, which is often overshadowed by more common gastrointestinal illnesses.

Even though it is frequently underestimated, the statistical prevalence of achalasia is quite important when it comes to chronic disorders. According to epidemiological studies, the prevalence is larger than previously thought, dispelling myths and highlighting the critical need for a thorough grasp of Achalasia's statistical footprint.

The demographic and geographic peculiarities of Achalasia, in addition to its prevalence, highlight the condition's complex aspects. Variations in incidence among age groups, genders, and ethnic groups highlight the complex interaction between environmental factors and genetic predispositions that shapes Achalasia's epidemiological landscape. We can develop customised solutions that cater to the specific needs of individuals in various demographics by gaining a comprehensive understanding of the various manifestations and implications of Achalasia via the deciphering of these demographic complexities.

Beyond its occurrence, Achalasia has a statistical background that affects quality of life, healthcare utilisation, and economic costs. People dealing with Achalasia frequently experience misdiagnoses, long wait times for proper care, and delayed diagnosis. Complicating matters, Achalasia's statistical underrepresentation makes it difficult to identify the condition in a timely manner and implement the customised interventions that are necessary to lessen its negative effects on people's quality of life.

Achalasia's statistical characteristics also highlight differences in the distribution of healthcare resources and access to specialist care, highlighting the need for patient-centered and equitable approaches that meet the unmet needs of those impacted by this chronic condition. The statistical frequency of Achalasia highlights the urgent need for comprehensive management techniques that include epidemiological insights into the care continuum and invites critical thought on the wider sociocultural and healthcare consequences.

Understanding the prevalence, patterns, and drivers of Achalasia is crucial, and epidemiological research lays a strong basis for well-informed decision-making and focused interventions that address the complex aspects of this esophageal motility condition. By illuminating the statistical facts surrounding Achalasia, we open the door to a life-changing experience that equips people, medical professionals, and legislators with the information and resources they need to successfully negotiate the complexity of this mysterious illness.

We explore the unexplored statistical terrain of Achalasia as we set out on this epidemiological journey, revealing important discoveries and answers that go beyond the boundaries of conventional healthcare narratives. A paradigm shift in our approach to comprehensive Achalasia therapy is required due to the far-reaching ramifications of the statistical prevalence of Achalasia, which is often overshadowed by more common gastrointestinal illnesses.

To sum up, the investigation of Achalasia from an epidemiological perspective is a crucial first step towards comprehending the statistical facts and consequences of this mysterious illness. Through our analysis of Achalasia's prevalence, demographic subtleties, and societal ramifications, we establish a solid basis for effectively negotiating its intricacies.

Diagnosis and Assessment

Recognizing the Signs: When to Seek Help

This chapter's goal is to inform readers about the early warning signs and symptoms of achalasia, which should compel them to seek medical attention. By the time this chapter ends, the reader will have a thorough awareness of the signs that call for medical attention from a specialist.

The objective of identifying the symptoms of Achalasia can be accomplished without the need for any particular supplies or conditions. Nonetheless, it would be helpful to have a fundamental grasp of the digestive system of humans as well as knowledge of the typical symptoms connected to gastrointestinal illnesses.

Understanding the symptoms of Achalasia in its entirety is necessary to recognise the condition's warning indications. Being conscious of the altered swallowing habits, chest pain, and other associated symptoms is the first step in this process. Early detection of these symptoms is essential in order to seek timely medical evaluation and assistance.

1. An alteration in swallowing habits is among the first indications of achalasia. Some people may experience trouble swallowing solid food, necessitating the use of liquids to facilitate food passage via the oesophagus. It is important to pay attention to this uncomfortable feeling of food being lodged in the throat or chest.

2. Achalasia may be indicated by chronic chest pain or discomfort, particularly after eating. This sensation is frequently characterised as a tightness or pressure in the chest, and it might be misdiagnosed as a heart condition. In order to receive the proper medical attention, it is essential to distinguish between symptoms of Achalasia and chest pain associated to a heart attack.

3. People who have achalasia may regurgitate undigested food, frequently accompanied by a burning feeling in the throat or chest.

If left untreated, this regurgitation can happen both during and after meals, causing severe discomfort and possibly nutritional deficits.

4. Because achalasia makes it difficult to eat enough food, it might cause unintentional weight loss. Reduced food intake, regurgitation, and trouble swallowing can all contribute to a slow but significant loss of body weight. It's critical to keep an eye on weight fluctuations and recognise any unexplained weight loss in order to rule out any underlying medical issues, like Achalasia.

5. People with advanced Achalasia may have respiratory symptoms including recurring pneumonia, aspiration, or coughing. The regurgitation of food and drinks into the airways causes these respiratory problems and increases the risk of aspiration pneumonia and other respiratory complications.

- Keeping a log of symptoms is crucial. It is important to note the occurrence and intensity of dysphagia, chest pain, regurgitation, and any related weight fluctuations. When diagnosing a patient, medical experts may find useful information in this record.

- Early medical examination is essential to stopping Achalasia from progressing further and minimising any problems. Postponing medical care might exacerbate symptoms and lower general health.

- People should refrain from self-medicating with over-the-counter medications for heartburn or stomach discomfort if their symptoms are ongoing or getting worse. These symptoms could be a sign of underlying diseases such achalasia, which would need to be evaluated and treated by a specialist physician.

As soon as Achalasia signs and symptoms are identified, a full range of diagnostic tests must be performed, such as barium swallow studies, esophageal manometry, and even endoscopic examinations. These tests are crucial for determining the proper course of treatment and verifying the existence of achalasia.

People should see primary care physicians or gastroenterologists for referrals if they are having trouble getting in contact with specialists or diagnostic institutions. Furthermore, being transparent with medical professionals on the particular symptoms encountered might hasten the diagnostic procedure and guarantee prompt action.

To sum up, identifying the symptoms of achalasia is an essential first step toward obtaining the right kind of medical attention. Individuals can enhance overall health outcomes by proactively addressing potential difficulties connected to Achalasia by being aware of the early warning signs and symptoms described in this chapter. To effectively manage Achalasia, it is critical to stay alert and sensitive to any changes in swallowing patterns, chest discomfort, or related symptoms. Early detection and action are crucial.

The Role of the Primary Care Physician

The primary care physician plays a crucial role in aiding the initial identification and referral process for suspected patients in the comprehensive therapy of Achalasia. The purpose of this chapter is to clarify the roles and contributions that primary care physicians play in recognising and promptly referring patients who exhibit symptoms suggestive of Achalasia, therefore accelerating the process of diagnosis and the development of treatment plans.

The primary care physician is a medical expert who is trained to provide comprehensive and ongoing care for a wide range of medical disorders. They frequently serve as the initial point of contact for those seeking medical attention. Their areas of specialisation include health promotion, preventive care, and the preliminary assessment and treatment of common health issues.

Primary care physicians are essential in identifying the early warning signs and symptoms of Achalasia, which might first manifest as generalised stomach discomfort or trouble swallowing. Primary care physicians can identify potential red flags indicative of underlying esophageal motility issues, including Achalasia, by doing a comprehensive history and physical examination. They are also in charge of organising the proper referrals to diagnostic centres and gastroenterologists for additional assessment and diagnosis confirmation.

The idea of primary care has changed over ages, coinciding with the shifting dynamics of healthcare delivery and the growing importance of preventive and holistic treatment, even though it is not immediately applicable in the present situation. Comprehending the developmental trajectory of primary care highlights its ongoing importance within the healthcare system.

Beyond simply diagnosing symptoms, the primary care physician has a more comprehensive role in managing Achalasia. It includes creating a cooperative network with radiologists, gastroenterologists, and other experts to guarantee prompt and efficient access to subspecialty care and diagnostic procedures. Primary care physicians facilitate the effective management of patients by integrating their practises within a larger multidisciplinary care framework. This helps patients navigate the intricate diagnostic and therapy paths that are specific to Achalasia.

Imagine the following situation: a patient complains to their primary care physician about persistent chest pain and occasional dysphagia. With an understanding of esophageal motility problems, the primary care physician does a comprehensive evaluation and may suspect Achalasia. The doctor then quickly makes a referral to a gastroenterologist to do additional assessment, which speeds up the diagnostic procedure and ultimately the start of focused treatment plans.

There is a prevalent misperception about the job of the primary care physician, which is that their involvement is just in treating common primary care illnesses. Nonetheless, primary care physicians play a critical role as gatekeepers when it comes to complicated disorders like Achalasia, starting the diagnostic process and allowing prompt referrals for specialised care.

Since patients with early Achalasia symptoms frequently visit their primary care physician, the latter's keen observation of possible warning signs and accelerated referral procedures have a substantial impact on how the patient's diagnostic journey unfolds and how quickly they can receive specialised care. Thus, the primary care physician's first identification and referral of suspected instances of Achalasia has significant consequences for prompt management and the best possible outcomes for the patient.

The primary care physician's job description encompasses not only diagnosing symptoms but also helping patients comprehend and become aware of the possible significance of those symptoms. Primary care physicians facilitate a collaborative approach to early identification and management of Achalasia by empowering individuals to actively participate in their healthcare journey through patient education and counselling.

Esophageal Motility Disorders

A range of illnesses known as esophageal motility disorders are defined by abnormal or compromised esophageal motility, which can result in symptoms such as regurgitation and difficulty swallowing. These conditions may impact the lower esophageal sphincter's relaxation, the esophagus's peristaltic function, or both, which may lead to a variety of clinical presentations.

In order to identify the various clinical presentations of esophageal motility disorders and to customise the right diagnostic and treatment approaches, it is imperative to comprehend the pathophysiology of these conditions. In order to provide prompt intervention and specialised care, primary care physicians should be skilled in identifying the subtle changes in symptomatology and clinical findings that may point to the presence of esophageal motility disorders, including Achalasia.

The early anatomists and physiologists' groundbreaking work laid the groundwork for modern understandings of esophageal function and dysmotility, and this understanding of esophageal motility disorders has evolved historically. This historical background emphasises the ongoing effort to decipher the intricate details of esophageal physiology and disease.

Within the larger context of gastrointestinal health, esophageal motility abnormalities are closely associated with illnesses including functional dyspepsia, eosinophilic esophagitis, and gastroesophageal reflux disease (GERD). Understanding how esophageal motility disorders interact with other gastrointestinal illnesses enables a thorough evaluation of patients presenting with non-specific digestive symptoms, which in turn enables early detection and focused treatment.

Think about a patient who comes to their primary care physician with a history of chest pain and occasional dysphagia. Based on the distinctive symptomatology and clinical findings, the primary care physician uses a thorough evaluation to determine whether esophageal motility problems may be present. The timely diagnosis and beginning of customised management for the underlying esophageal motility issue is made possible by a subsequent referral to a gastroenterologist for expert evaluation and esophageal function tests.

One common misperception about esophageal motility problems is that they are caused by harmless factors like ageing or food preferences. This can cause symptoms to go undiagnosed and untreated. In order to avoid potential diagnostic delays and problems, primary care physicians are essential in dispelling these myths. They advocate for a complete evaluation and investigation of esophageal motility disorders in persons who present with suggestive symptoms.

The ability of primary care physicians to identify esophageal motility abnormalities and promptly send patients for specialised evaluation is crucial for streamlining the diagnostic process and guaranteeing focused treatment as they negotiate the complex terrain of patient care. Primary care physicians support the cornerstone of patient-centered care by taking a holistic approach to early recognition and referral, which improves the overall quality of care for patients with suspected esophageal motility problems.

Barium Swallow Studies

Barium swallow studies, sometimes referred to as esophagrams, are diagnostic imaging techniques that involve radiographic viewing of the oesophagus after the administration of barium contrast material. The evaluation of esophageal morphology, motility, and functional abnormalities made possible by these investigations offers important new information about the existence of structural or functional esophageal diseases, such as achalasia.

Barium swallow tests provide dynamic imaging of esophageal peristalsis, esophagogastric junction relaxation, and the presence of esophageal outflow obstruction, making them a fundamental diagnostic tool for esophageal motility disorders. In order to determine the underlying pathophysiology of suspected esophageal motility disorders and to inform subsequent referral and management methods, primary care physicians should be aware of the value of barium swallow examinations.

Barium swallow studies have a long history that began with the early use of barium-based contrast agents in gastrointestinal radiography, which transformed esophageal visibility and led to important advances in our knowledge of esophageal illnesses. This historical background emphasises the continued value of barium swallow examinations as a diagnostic tool for illnesses involving the motility of the oesophagus.

Barium swallow studies interact with modalities like esophageal manometry and endoscopy to assess esophageal function and pathology in a complete manner. They are placed within the larger context of diagnostic radiography and functional imaging. Acknowledging the supplementary function of barium swallow examinations in the diagnostic algorithm for illnesses pertaining to esophageal motility improves the comprehensive evaluation of individuals exhibiting suggestive symptoms, thus enabling focused treatment and attention.

Imagine a patient who has a history of regurgitation and dysphagia and who visits their primary care provider. The primary care physician schedules a barium swallow examination to evaluate the structure and function of the oesophagus in light of the possible suspicion of esophageal motility problems. When the ensuing radiographic results show traits suggestive of Achalasia, a gastroenterologist is consulted immediately for additional testing and customised care.

One widespread misperception about barium swallow studies is that they are only thought of as anatomical imaging studies, ignoring the dynamic evaluation of esophageal motility and functional problems that they provide. Dispelling these myths is a major responsibility of primary care physicians, who support the extensive use of barium swallow examinations to identify the underlying pathophysiology of esophageal motility disorders. This allows for prompt referral and focused management.

Understanding the critical role barium swallow studies play in revealing esophageal pathology and directing subsequent management is crucial for primary care physicians as they navigate the diagnostic evaluation of patients with suspected esophageal motility disorders. This helps to expedite the diagnostic process and guarantee the best possible care. Through

Advanced Diagnostic Techniques

During the diagnostic process for Achalasia, the application of sophisticated diagnostic methods is essential for verifying the existence of this esophageal motility problem and defining its particular features. The purpose of this chapter is to examine the specific diagnostic procedures used in the assessment of Achalasia, with an emphasis on the thorough comprehension and utilisation of barium swallow studies and esophageal manometry. Healthcare providers and those impacted by Achalasia can learn a great deal about the complex diagnostic environment around this disorder by understanding the guiding principles, indications, and interpretive subtleties of these diagnostic modalities.

Esophageal manometry is a vital component of the diagnostic toolkit for Achalasia since it provides a dynamic evaluation of the lower esophageal sphincter's function and esophageal motility. By inserting a catheter equipped with pressure sensors into the oesophagus, this approach allows for the accurate assessment of esophageal motility coordination, relaxation of the lower esophageal sphincter, and esophageal peristalsis. Esophageal manometry provides vital insights into the pathophysiology of Achalasia by carefully examining the pressure patterns and contractile strength of the oesophagus. This allows for the diagnosis and distinction of Achalasia from other esophageal motility disorders.

Barium swallow tests, or esophagrams, are a crucial part of the Achalasia diagnostic protocol because they offer radiographic visualisation of the architecture, motility, and functional problems of the oesophagus. This diagnostic technique entails ingesting barium contrast material, which is then followed by dynamic radiography imaging to detect esophageal outflow blockage, esophagogastric junction relaxation, and esophageal peristalsis. Through the identification of distinctive radiographic characteristics, barium swallow investigations aid in the final confirmation and clinical categorization of this intricate esophageal motility condition.

Think about a patient who comes to their gastroenterologist with a long history of dysphagia, regurgitation, and chest pain. When a gastroenterologist suspects esophageal motility abnormalities, they schedule an extensive evaluation that includes esophageal manometry. Aperistalsis and reduced lower esophageal sphincter relaxation are visible in the recorded pressure tracings, which are in line with the Achalasia diagnosis. The radiographic evidence of esophageal outflow obstruction is further supported by a subsequent referral for barium swallow investigations, which confirms the diagnosis and directs the patient's individualised treatment plan.

From a clinical perspective, the use of barium swallow tests and esophageal manometry goes beyond simple diagnostic confirmation and includes the phenotypic categorization and prognostication of Achalasia. Healthcare professionals can categorise Achalasia into different subgroups, each with its own treatment implications and prognosis factors, by identifying the specific manometric patterns and radiographic findings. Healthcare practitioners can optimise patient outcomes and quality of life by customising tailored management approaches with the support of a thorough understanding of various diagnostic techniques.

Furthermore, the patient may experience anxiety and uncertainty when negotiating the complexities of barium swallow examinations and esophageal manometry. Healthcare professionals can reduce patient fear and encourage active participation in the diagnostic process by clarifying the procedure specifics, anticipated feelings, and possible results of these tests. Giving those impacted by Achalasia the information and comprehension of these diagnostic techniques fosters a team-based approach to treatment, fortifying the relationship between patients and providers and improving the diagnostic process as a whole.

With over 90% diagnostic accuracy in confirming the diagnosis of Achalasia, esophageal manometry plays a crucial role in providing a clear description of this esophageal motility condition. Furthermore, the development of high-resolution esophageal manometry has transformed the accuracy and interpretive breadth of this diagnostic technique, making it possible to distinguish minute pressure fluctuations and esophageal motor patterns that are suggestive of Achalasia subtypes.

Barium swallow investigations, on the other hand, have a sensitivity and specificity of over 80% in identifying esophageal motility problems, such as Achalasia, highlighting its critical function in radiographic evaluation and conclusive confirmation of this condition. When combined with the evaluation of esophageal outflow dynamics, the dynamic visualisation of barium transit through the oesophagus offers vital radiographic evidence that is crucial to the thorough definition of Achalasia and its phenotypic subgroups.

A tiny catheter with pressure sensors is inserted into the oesophagus during esophageal manometry, which is sometimes thought of as a difficult and involved diagnostic procedure. This allows for the accurate assessment of esophageal peristalsis and lower esophageal sphincter function. Esophageal manometry, through a thorough assessment of the pressure dynamics and contractile strength of the oesophagus, outlines the distinct motor patterns and relaxation traits characteristic of Achalasia and its subtypes.

On the other hand, barium swallow studies are a non-invasive and useful diagnostic technique for Achalasia, even if they need the intake of barium contrast material and dynamic radiography imaging. The radiographic evidence that is vital for verifying the diagnostic and phenotypic classification of Achalasia is provided by the visualisation of barium transit through the oesophagus and the evaluation of esophageal outflow dynamics.

In summary, a thorough comprehension and utilisation of barium swallow tests and esophageal manometry are essential elements in the diagnostic assessment of achalasia. By carefully evaluating esophageal motility, pressure dynamics, and radiographic features, these sophisticated diagnostic methods confirm the existence of Achalasia and clarify its underlying pathophysiology, allowing for the development of customised treatment plans and prognosis factors. These diagnostic modalities uphold the cornerstone of patient-centered care by encouraging a collaborative approach between healthcare providers and individuals affected by Achalasia. This approach optimises diagnostic accuracy and improves the overall quality of care for this complex esophageal motility disorder.

Misdiagnosis: Common Pitfalls and Prevention

Raising awareness of the widespread problem of misdiagnoses is crucial as we negotiate the complex terrain of managing achalasia. Misdiagnoses can trap both individuals and medical professionals. Misdiagnoses of Achalasia provide a significant challenge in the proper and early identification of this ailment, since they frequently result from overlapping symptomatology with other esophageal conditions. This chapter aims to analyse the typical errors that result in incorrect diagnoses, explore the possible ramifications of these errors, and outline preventative measures to strengthen the diagnostic process in order to protect the health of those who are dealing with Achalasia.

The main problem here is that Achalasia is presented in a complex and frequently cryptic way that makes it easy to misunderstand and misclassify. Though characteristic of Achalasia, the typical symptoms of dysphagia, regurgitation, and chest tightness also coexist with a variety of esophageal and non-esophageal illnesses, complicating the diagnosis. As a result, medical professionals could unintentionally ignore the subtleties unique to Achalasia, leading to incorrect diagnosis and treatment diversion.

Misdiagnosing Achalasia can have a wide range of consequences that affect patients and healthcare systems in significant ways. From a patient perspective, long-term diagnostic journeys, significant emotional anguish, and a delay in starting specialised treatment plans are caused by the mismatch between the accepted diagnosis and the underlying pathophysiology of Achalasia. Moreover, the unintentional use of improper interventions based on misdiagnoses not only increases the severity of symptoms but also raises the risk of iatrogenic repercussions, which lowers the quality of life for those who are dealing with Achalasia.

The financial fallout from incorrect diagnoses is felt systemically, as the resources and infrastructure of healthcare are depleted by repeated rounds of unproductive tests, consultations, and investigations. Long-term diagnostic paths caused by incorrect diagnoses prolong healthcare delivery inefficiencies and foster a climate of apprehension and disillusionment among patients and healthcare professionals alike.

Given these challenges, a multifaceted strategy that is based on a careful balancing act between clinical expertise, investigative accuracy, and patient-centered awareness becomes the front-runner in the fight against incorrect diagnosis of Achalasia. Preventing misdiagnoses is largely dependent on the use of sophisticated diagnostic techniques and their ability to discriminatively untangle the complexities of esophageal motility. Simultaneously, it is critical to strengthen diagnostic acumen by cultivating a climate of active communication and knowledge sharing between patients and healthcare providers, as well as a persistent attention in examining the nuances of symptomatology.

To implement these ideas, the diagnostic paradigm must be rethought in a way that is based on a comprehensive understanding of the clinical, radiographic, and manometric symptoms of Achalasia. Physicians are advised to reevaluate their diagnostic criteria and adopt a higher threshold of suspicion for Achalasia among the range of esophageal diseases. The cornerstone of an extensive diagnostic arsenal is the prudent combination of esophageal manometry, high-resolution esophageal pressure topography, and functional luminal imaging probe tests, supported by thorough symptom profiling and nutritional evaluation.

At the same time, providing those impacted by Achalasia with a clear comprehension of the primary symptoms, diagnostic tests, and possible differentials empowers patients and healthcare professionals to work together to create a cooperative environment that is favourable to identifying the true diagnosis amidst the diagnostic maze.

It is predicted that the adoption of these preventative approaches will result in a multitude of benefits, which can be viewed through the lenses of improved patient outcomes, simpler treatment plans, and increased diagnostic accuracy. With the support of cutting-edge modalities and a sophisticated understanding of esophageal motility disorders, the diagnostic pathways will be strengthened, significantly reducing the risk of misdiagnosis and paving the way for a new era of therapeutic efficacy and diagnostic accuracy.

Furthermore, a symbiotic patient-provider alliance can be fostered through the development of an informed and involved patient cohort, which is supported by a deliberate effort to simplify the diagnostic process and create an atmosphere of shared decision-making. Consequently, it is expected that this will enhance patient compliance, maximise treatment adherence, and produce a noticeable improvement in the general health and standard of living for those coping with the unpredictable nature of Achalasia.

Although the identified solutions form the cornerstone of a strong defence against misdiagnoses of Achalasia, it is necessary to recognise the supplementary function of interdisciplinary teams and the prudent application of supplemental investigative techniques in strengthening the diagnostic journey. The smooth collaboration of radiologists, thoracic surgeons, and gastroenterologists along with the incorporation of additional diagnostic instruments like impedance studies and esophageal pH monitoring could enhance diagnostic knowledge, solve diagnostic puzzles, and avoid misdiagnosis traps.

To sum up, stopping and preventing misdiagnoses of Achalasia requires a coordinated effort based on three key elements: accurate diagnosis, active patient participation, and multidisciplinary teamwork. By carefully incorporating these principles into the clinical setting, the diagnostic journey will be strengthened against the unpredictable nature of incorrect diagnoses, leading to a paradigm change in the treatment of Achalasia that is supported by both therapeutic efficacy and diagnostic fidelity.

The Patient's Role in Diagnosis

This chapter's main goal is to empower people who are attempting to navigate the complex world of Achalasia diagnosis by highlighting the critical role that the patient plays in the diagnostic process. The reader will receive the cognitive scaffolding required to navigate their diagnostic trip with resilience and perspicacity by clarifying the key concepts of self-advocacy, informed consent, and active involvement in the ordeal.

The reader is advised to prepare for this enlightening journey by preparing an open mind, a strong dedication to their health, and a voracious appetite for information. Furthermore, making the most of this chapter requires assimilating basic knowledge regarding the primary symptoms of Achalasia, the diagnostic modalities pertinent to its clarification, and the possible differentials that could complicate the diagnosis process.

The trip begins with a broad overview of the natural partnership that exists between patients and healthcare professionals, based on a mutual dedication to figuring out the diagnostic puzzle that surrounds Achalasia. This symbiotic relationship, which is anchored on respect for one another, candid communication, and joint decision-making, creates an atmosphere that is favourable to accurate diagnosis and successful treatment. The chapter then unfolds a step-by-step plan outlining the critical role that patients play in the diagnostic environment, culminating in the development of a knowledgeable and capable patient population that is ready to overcome the diagnostic dead ends that confront Achalasia.

The core of patient empowerment in the diagnostic domain is based on a steadfast dedication to self-advocacy, which is supported by a clear understanding of the primary symptoms of Achalasia and the diagnostic techniques that aid in its diagnosis. People are encouraged to cultivate an atmosphere of candid communication with their medical professionals, clearly and precisely expressing their symptomatology. When a thorough symptom diary, which carefully documents the subtleties of dysphagia, regurgitation, and chest pain, is carefully combined with a critical evaluation of dietary preferences and aggravating factors, it provides physicians with critical information that is essential to accelerating the diagnosis process.

At the same time, people are encouraged to get a thorough knowledge of the diagnostic tools available to them, which include barium esophagography, esophageal manometry, high-resolution esophageal pressure topography, and functional luminal imaging probe studies. Through gaining a basic understanding of the complexities underlying these diagnostic modalities, people are better equipped to converse with their healthcare providers, understand the reasoning behind diagnostic studies, and take part in the collaborative decision-making environment that forms the basis of the diagnostic journey.

People are advised to proceed through the diagnostic maze of Achalasia with an unyielding sense of thoroughness and an unbreakable spirit of resistance. The core principles of self-advocacy are inextricably linked to a dedication to strengthening one's knowledge base, being aware of the diagnostic modalities and their significance, and being honest and straightforward when expressing one's symptomatology. However, people are warned about the dangers of giving in to the allure of diagnostic self-attribution, in which assimilating fragmented knowledge leads to an increased likelihood of incorrect diagnostic attributions and excessive anxiety.

In addition, people are urged to be aware of the possible traps that could entangle the diagnosis procedure due to Achalasia's overlapping symptomatology with a variety of esophageal and non-esophageal illnesses. The combination of symptoms could confuse the path of diagnosis, requiring a careful evaluation of the subtleties unique to

Achalasia and its differentials to prevent misdiagnosis and unnecessary treatment paths.

The implementation of patient empowerment principles in the diagnostic setting requires the presence of a well-informed and actively participating patient population that is seamlessly woven into the diagnostic fabric. The tangible improvement in the diagnostic trajectory, the prompt diagnosis of Achalasia, and the development of a cooperative patient-provider relationship based on respect and collaborative decision-making serve as evidence that this paradigm change is valid.

Should a patient experience diagnostic dead ends or unclear diagnoses, they are urged to engage in candid communication with their physicians and push for a thorough reassessment of their diagnostic path. Bringing together a multidisciplinary team consisting of radiologists, thoracic surgeons, and gastroenterologists could be helpful in solving diagnostic puzzles, avoiding false positives, and fostering diagnostic integrity.

In summary, the patient now plays a more active role in the diagnostic process than just a passive recipient, strengthening the diagnostic process with a combination of informed consent, self-advocacy, and a cooperative patient-provider partnership. This convergence, which is based on the principles of respect for one another and collaborative decision-making, creates a diagnostic environment that is accurate, proactive, and effective in treatment, thereby permanently changing the fabric of Achalasia care.

Interpreting Test Results: A Guide for Patients

For patients navigating the complexity of managing their health, it is critical that they comprehend the terminology and jargon involved with diagnostic test results. Patients are able to ask knowledgeable questions, take an active role in their care, and decide on their course of treatment because to this understanding. This chapter seeks to provide patients the means to grasp their test results by emphasising important terms that are critical to comprehending the material and connecting them to practical ideas. This will help patients feel more in charge of their care and more like partners in it.

In order to facilitate a comprehensive understanding of diagnostic test results, it is imperative to define and elucidate a multitude of terms that are pertinent to the diagnostic process. These terms include but are not limited to:

1. Sensitivity
2. Specificity
3. Positive predictive value
4. Negative predictive value
5. Accuracy
6. Precision
7. True positive
8. True negative
9. False positive
10. False negative
11. Confidence interval
12. Reference range
13. Standard deviation
14. Medical terminology specific to the diagnostic test being discussed

1. Sensitivity:

The capacity of a diagnostic test to accurately identify people who have the condition of interest is known as sensitivity. A test with high sensitivity will accurately detect a significant number of people with the illness, reducing the number of false negative results.

2. Specificity:

The capacity of a diagnostic test to accurately identify people who do not have the ailment of interest is referred to as specificity. A highly specific test will reduce false positives by accurately ruling out people who do not have the illness.

3. Positive Predictive Value:

The percentage of real positive results among all positive results is known as the test's positive predictive value. It indicates the likelihood that a positive test result actually reflects the existence of the ailment.

4. Negative Predictive Value:

The percentage of real negative results among all negative results is known as the test's negative predictive value. It sheds light on the likelihood that a negative test result actually signifies the illness is absent.

5. Accuracy:

How closely the test findings match the actual value is shown in accuracy. It provides a comprehensive assessment of the test's performance, taking into account both sensitivity and specificity.

6. Precision:

Reproducibility of test results is what is meant by precision. Repeating a precise test with the same parameters will produce consistent results.

7. True Positive:

When a test accurately detects the ailment in a person who actually has it, the result is deemed to be true positive.

8. True Negative:

When a test accurately detects the absence of a condition in a person who actually does not have it, the result is a genuine negative.

9. False Positive:

When a test falsely detects the presence of a condition in a person who does not genuinely have it, the result is referred to as a false positive.

10. False Negative:

When a test falsely reveals that a person does not have a condition when in fact they do, this is known as a false negative result.

11. Confidence Interval:

The range of values that a confidence interval offers indicates how likely it is that the true value will fall. It shows how accurate the estimate that was made using the sample data was.

12. Reference Range:

The reference range is the range of values that, in a healthy population, is regarded as typical for a particular test. Generally speaking, results that fall inside this range are regarded as normal.

13. Standard Deviation:

A set of values' degree of variation or dispersion is measured by its standard deviation. It sheds light on how widely apart the data points are from the mean.

14. Medical Terminology Specific to the Diagnostic Test:

Depending on the nature of the diagnostic test, there may be specific medical terminology and jargon that patients should be familiar with in order to interpret their results accurately. This may include terms related to imaging studies, laboratory tests, or other specialized diagnostic modalities.

To facilitate a deeper understanding of these terms, it can be helpful to connect them to real-world scenarios or familiar concepts. For instance, consider the concept of sensitivity and specificity in the context of a security screening process at an airport. A highly sensitive security system would detect nearly all prohibited items, ensuring that very few dangerous items are missed (minimizing false negatives). On the other hand, a highly specific security system would accurately identify only prohibited items, minimizing the occurrence of false alarms (minimizing false positives).

Similarly, the positive predictive value and negative predictive value can be likened to the accuracy of weather forecasts. A high positive predictive value is akin to a weather forecast that accurately predicts rain when rain is indeed on the horizon, while a high negative predictive value is akin to a forecast that accurately predicts clear skies when no rain is expected.

By drawing parallels to familiar concepts, patients can grasp the nuances of these technical terms more readily, empowering them to interpret their test results with greater confidence and understanding.

Case Study: A Diagnostic Journey

Sarah, a 35-year-old woman, had been experiencing persistent difficulty in swallowing for several months. Initially, she attributed it to stress and anxiety, assuming that her symptoms were a manifestation of her hectic lifestyle. However, as the problem persisted and worsened, she sought medical attention. Sarah's journey from the onset of her symptoms to the confirmation of her diagnosis of Achalasia offers valuable insights into the challenges faced by patients with esophageal motility disorders and the strategies employed to address these issues.

Sarah, the protagonist of this case study, is a vibrant and determined individual who leads a busy life as a marketing executive. Her commitment to her career and her passion for travel and exploring new cuisines are central aspects of her identity. As she grappled with the distressing symptoms of dysphagia and regurgitation, she sought the expertise of Dr. Ankita Kashyap, a medical doctor with a holistic approach to healthcare and a focus on empowering patients to actively participate in their well-being. Under Dr. Kashyap's guidance, Sarah embarked on a diagnostic journey that ultimately led to the identification of her condition and the initiation of a comprehensive management plan.

The core challenge that Sarah faced was the accurate identification and understanding of her symptoms, a task compounded by the subtle and insidious nature of Achalasia. The progressive nature of the condition and its overlap with common digestive complaints posed a diagnostic conundrum, necessitating a meticulous approach to unravel the underlying cause of Sarah's distress. Additionally, the impact of her symptoms on her quality of life and emotional well-being underscored the urgency of addressing this challenge effectively.

Dr. Kashyap and her team initiated a comprehensive diagnostic process, encompassing a thorough medical history, a detailed physical examination, and a series of specialized tests tailored to assess esophageal motility and function. Sarah underwent a barium swallow study, esophageal manometry, and upper endoscopy, each offering distinct insights into the dynamics of her esophageal function. These modalities, in conjunction with a patient-centered approach that emphasized active communication and collaboration, formed the cornerstone of the diagnostic strategy.

The culmination of the diagnostic evaluation revealed characteristic findings consistent with Achalasia, elucidating the pathophysiological basis of Sarah's symptoms. This definitive diagnosis provided clarity and validation for Sarah, affirming the legitimacy of her experiences and paving the way for targeted interventions. The subsequent formulation of a personalized management plan, integrating dietary modifications, behavioral strategies, and potential therapeutic interventions, marked a pivotal milestone in Sarah's journey towards comprehensive achalasia management.

The case of Sarah illuminates the intricate interplay between patient experiences and diagnostic challenges in the realm of esophageal motility disorders. It underscores the imperative of a patient-centric approach to healthcare, wherein active engagement and partnership with patients serve as catalysts for accurate diagnosis and effective management. Furthermore, the case exemplifies the significance of interdisciplinary collaboration and the integration of holistic healthcare modalities in addressing the multifaceted dimensions of achalasia and its impact on patients' lives.

Incorporating graphical representations of the diagnostic tests and anatomical illustrations of the esophagus would enhance the reader's understanding of the investigative process and the anatomical aberrations characteristic of Achalasia.

Sarah's journey serves as a microcosm of the broader narrative surrounding the diagnostic odyssey of patients with esophageal motility disorders. The insights gleaned from her experience resonate with the overarching theme of patient empowerment and the pivotal role of interdisciplinary collaboration in navigating the complexities of achalasia management. By contextualizing the nuances of Sarah's case within the broader landscape of esophageal health, the case study underscores the need for continued dialogue and research to optimize diagnostic pathways and therapeutic approaches for individuals grappling with achalasia.

As we delve deeper into the intricate tapestry of achalasia management, a fundamental question emerges: How can the convergence of patient advocacy, medical expertise, and holistic wellness philosophies synergistically inform the design of tailored management strategies for achalasia and other esophageal motility disorders?

As Dr. Ankita Kashyap continues to guide her patients through the intricate terrain of achalasia management, the case of Sarah stands as a testament to the transformative potential of patient-centric healthcare and the unyielding pursuit of comprehensive wellness.

Treatment Options

Pharmacological Interventions: Medications and Beyond

In the management of achalasia, pharmacological interventions play a crucial role in alleviating symptoms and improving esophageal function. Understanding the current medications used, their mechanisms of action, and their specific roles in symptom control is essential for developing a comprehensive approach to achalasia management. In this chapter, we will explore the pharmacological interventions for achalasia, delving into the mechanisms of action, evidence supporting their use, and their practical applications in clinical settings.

1. Calcium Channel Blockers
2. Nitrates
3. Botulinum Toxin Injections
4. Phosphodiesterase-5 Inhibitors
5. Anticholinergic Medications
6. Endothelin Receptor Antagonists

Calcium channel blockers, such as nifedipine and verapamil, are commonly used in the management of achalasia due to their ability to relax smooth muscle in the esophagus. These medications inhibit the influx of calcium ions into the smooth muscle cells, leading to vasodilation and decreased muscle contractility. The relaxation of the lower esophageal sphincter (LES) and esophageal smooth muscle results in improved bolus transit and reduced dysphagia in patients with achalasia.

The mechanism of action of calcium channel blockers involves blocking L-type calcium channels in the smooth muscle cells of the esophagus. By inhibiting calcium influx, these medications reduce the contractility of the esophageal smooth muscle, leading to relaxation of the LES and esophageal body. This relaxation facilitates the passage of food and liquids through the esophagus, addressing the dysphagia and regurgitation associated with achalasia.

Clinical studies have demonstrated the efficacy of calcium channel blockers in improving dysphagia and esophageal function in patients with achalasia. Research has shown that nifedipine, in particular, can significantly reduce LES pressure and improve esophageal emptying, leading to symptomatic relief in a substantial proportion of patients. Furthermore, patient testimonials often highlight the relief of dysphagia and regurgitation following the initiation of calcium channel blocker therapy.

In clinical practice, calcium channel blockers are often prescribed as a first-line pharmacological intervention for achalasia, especially in patients who are not candidates for more invasive treatments. These medications offer a non-invasive approach to symptom management and can be particularly beneficial for patients with mild to moderate achalasia symptoms. However, it is important to monitor for potential side effects, such as hypotension and headache, and adjust the dosage accordingly to optimize therapeutic benefits.

Having elucidated the mechanisms and practical considerations of calcium channel blockers, we now turn our attention to another class of medications used in the pharmacological management of achalasia: nitrates. By exploring the role of nitrates in esophageal relaxation and symptom control, we aim to provide a comprehensive understanding of the diverse pharmacological interventions available for achalasia management.

Endoscopic Procedures: A Minimally Invasive Approach

Endoscopic procedures are a good choice for patients who might not be good candidates for more invasive surgical therapies since they provide a minimally invasive method to treating achalasia. This chapter focuses on balloon dilation and peroral endoscopic myotomy in order to provide a thorough overview of the endoscopic techniques available for treating achalasia (POEM). Our aim is to offer a comprehensive understanding of the role that these methods play in managing achalasia by exploring their processes, supporting evidence, and useful applications.

Pneumatic dilation, another name for balloon dilation, is a minimally invasive endoscopic therapy that works to damage the muscle fibres that make up the lower esophageal sphincter (LES), lessening its hypertonicity and improving bolus transit in the oesophagus. An endoscope with a deflated balloon is inserted into the oesophagus and placed across the lower esophageal sphincter (LES) during the surgery. After positioning itself, the balloon is inflated to a preset pressure, applying radial strain to the LES and causing the muscle fibres to be deliberately disrupted.

The mechanical disruption of the LES muscle fibres is the main mechanism by which balloon dilation reduces sphincter pressure over time. By creating microtears in the smooth muscle due to the regulated radial tension applied by the inflated balloon, LES pressure is reduced and muscular relaxation is encouraged. In the end, this procedure helps individuals with achalasia with their dysphagia and esophageal emptying.

Take the example of a 45-year-old patient with type II achalasia who, in spite of conservative treatment, continues to experience dysphagia and regurgitation. Balloon dilation is scheduled for the patient after a gastroenterologist's evaluation. In order to disrupt the hypertonic LES, the balloon is inflated at a specific pressure while the endoscope is carefully placed into position during the surgery. The patient's dysphagia symptoms have significantly improved, according to follow-up appointments, which emphasises the effectiveness of balloon dilation in the treatment of achalasia.

Although balloon dilation has been shown to be effective in lowering LES pressure and enhancing dysphagia in achalasia patients, it is crucial to take into account any possible hazards and consequences. Research has indicated that there are positive short-term results from balloon dilation, with a significant number of patients reporting symptomatic alleviation. Long-term statistics, however, highlight the necessity for continuous monitoring and tailored treatment, as some patients may need repeat dilations due to symptom recurrence or inadequate response.

Clinical research has shed important light on the effectiveness of balloon dilatation in the treatment of achalasia. Pneumatic dilation has been demonstrated to significantly lower LES pressure and facilitate esophageal emptying, with positive results seen in cases of primary and recurring achalasia. Additionally, findings suggest that balloon dilation is a better alternative for some patient demographics than surgical myotomy due to reduced incidence of post-procedural problems.

Patients may not be familiar with several of the technical jargon and concepts used in the balloon dilation process. To improve comprehension, let me make it clear that pneumatic dilation is the process of using air pressure to expand a balloon inside the oesophagus, applying pressure to the LES in order to cause muscular disruption. The goal of this carefully timed interruption is to lessen the sphincter's hypertonicity, which will enhance esophageal function and alleviate symptoms in achalasia patients.

To sum up, balloon dilation is a minimally invasive endoscopic treatment that provides a useful therapy strategy for achalasia.

Healthcare professionals can successfully assist patients in making decisions by having a thorough understanding of the mechanism, supporting data, and useful considerations surrounding balloon dilation. This allows them to ensure that patients receive individualised treatment plans that maximise esophageal function and symptom relief.

For the treatment of achalasia, a novel and minimally invasive endoscopic technique called peroral endoscopic myotomy (POEM) has gained popularity. By creating a submucosal tunnel endoscopically and then myotomizing the esophageal muscle layers, this procedure specifically disrupts the LES and facilitates bolus transit into the oesophagus. The minimally invasive toolkit for managing achalasia has grown dramatically with the introduction of POEM, which presents a viable substitute for the more established surgical myotomy.

In order to access the muscle layers beneath the mucosa, POEM involves creating a submucosal tunnel in the oesophagus. After the tunnelling stage, a myotomy is carried out to specifically damage the LES's circular muscle fibres in order to gradually lower the sphincter pressure. This specific method addresses the functional impairment associated with achalasia by restoring esophageal peristalsis and improving bolus transit.

Discussions over POEM's safety, effectiveness, and relative advantages over conventional treatment approaches have been triggered by its debut. POEM proponents emphasise that their technique can accomplish targeted myotomy with minimal invasiveness, which may lower the risk of problems following surgery and expedite healing. To maximise the advantages of POEM in the management of achalasia, critics point out that long-term data on patient outcomes and thorough examination of patient selection criteria are necessary.

The literature that highlights POEM's safety profile and effectiveness has been increasing, adding to the body of evidence that supports its usage in the management of achalasia. Research has shown that POEM has positive short-term effects, including notable improvements in dysphagia, LES pressure, and esophageal emptying. With a low rate of procedure-related adverse effects and long-term data indicating continued symptomatic improvement, POEM appears to be a potential treatment for some achalasia patients.

In order to improve understanding of POEM, the technical details of the process must be made clear. Stressing to patients that a peroral endoscopic myotomy entails the formation of a submucosal tunnel in conjunction with a targeted myotomy of the LES muscle layers will help them comprehend the reasoning and methodology behind this minimally invasive procedure. Clarifying POEM's function in improving esophageal function and reducing dysphagia can also give patients the knowledge they need to make decisions about their course of treatment.

To sum up, peroral endoscopic myotomy is a major development in the least invasive treatment of achalasia, providing a customised strategy for LES disruption and restoration of esophageal function. Healthcare professionals can educate patients and involve them in conversations about individualised treatment plans by examining the theory, supporting data, and many points of view surrounding POEM. This will ultimately improve the quality of life and results for people with achalasia.

This chapter has covered endoscopic techniques for managing achalasia, with a particular emphasis on the less invasive balloon dilation and peroral endoscopic myotomy procedures (POEM). Through the clarification of the mechanisms, supporting data, and pragmatic factors related to these treatments, our goal is to offer healthcare professionals with the understanding and information required to assist patients in making decisions and carry out individualised treatment plans. To guarantee the best possible care for people with achalasia, it is essential to stay up to date on the most recent developments and research in the field of endoscopic interventions.

Surgical Solutions: When to Consider

Achalasia is a complex esophageal motility condition that causes dysphagia, regurgitation, chest discomfort, and weight loss. It is characterised by poor relaxation of the lower esophageal sphincter (LES) and missing peristalsis in the esophageal body. Even though endoscopic techniques like balloon dilation and peroral endoscopic myotomy (POEM) provide effective minimally invasive therapies for managing achalasia, surgical interventions are sometimes required. The purpose of this chapter is to examine the conditions that warrant surgical intervention for achalasia, including the kinds of procedures that can be performed and the anticipated results.

Even while endoscopic procedures are effective, certain achalasia patients may still require more final intervention due to ongoing symptoms or consequences. To optimise patient care and outcomes in the management of this difficult condition, it is essential to comprehend the particular conditions that call for surgical intervention.

Patients may suffer for an extended period of time if surgical intervention is not performed when it is necessary. This may include persistent dysphagia, malnourishment, aspiration pneumonia, and a decreased quality of life. Furthermore, postponing surgery when there are serious side effects like megaesophagus or esophageal cancer can worsen the condition and increase related morbidity.

Achalasia can be treated surgically using a variety of techniques, such as laparoscopic Heller myotomy, esophagectomy, and endoscopic anti-reflux operations. For patients with refractory or advanced achalasia, these surgical techniques attempt to disrupt the aberrant LES function, ease symptoms, and prevent esophageal problems. They also offer a long-lasting treatment.

When implementing surgical remedies for achalasia, a thorough assessment of patient-specific variables, such as symptom severity, esophageal function, comorbidities, and personalised treatment objectives, must be conducted. The best surgical technique is chosen with the help of this customised approach, which also makes it easier to prepare for and recover after surgery.

Research assessing the long-term consequences of achalasia surgery has shown promising outcomes, such as improved esophageal function, prolonged symptom alleviation, and improved quality of life. Moreover, improvements in perioperative care and surgical skill have led to lower rates of morbidity and better outcomes following surgery, which has increased the overall effectiveness of surgical treatments for achalasia.

Even though endoscopic procedures are often successful, there are some situations in which other surgical techniques, such as esophagectomy with or without reconstruction, might be taken into consideration. These situations are especially relevant for patients who have concurrent esophageal pathology or end-stage achalasia.

Surgical Guidelines and Pointers

When managing patients with achalasia, surgical options are taken into account when symptoms are severe, dysphagia returns after endoscopic procedures, esophageal problems emerge, or patients show up with advanced disease stages. It is crucial to comprehend the surgical intervention indications in order to handle achalasia promptly and effectively.

The decision to pursue surgical solutions in achalasia is guided by several clinical indicators, including:

- Refractory Symptoms: Patients who do not achieve adequate symptom relief with endoscopic procedures or experience recurrent dysphagia despite prior interventions may benefit from surgical evaluation.

- Esophageal Complications: To arrest the disease's progression and associated morbidity, surgical intervention may be required when severe esophageal stasis, megaesophagus, or esophageal dilatation emerge.

- Esophageal Malignancy: When achalasia is exacerbated by esophageal cancer, it is imperative to seek early surgical attention and treatment, which frequently entails esophagectomy along with lymphadenectomy.

A thorough evaluation is necessary to determine the extent of achalasia, examine esophageal function, and find any relevant comorbidities that might affect treatment choices before deciding on surgical intervention. Diagnostic tools such upper endoscopy, esophageal manometry, and esophagogram are essential for defining the features of the disease and helping determine the best surgical strategy.

Laparoscopic Heller Myotomy: 0Laparoscopic Heller myotomy, which is thought to be the gold standard surgical treatment for achalasia, involves the selective separation of the LES muscle fibres to relieve the functional blockage and facilitate esophageal emptying. Compared to the open myotomy procedure, this minimally invasive method has shorter hospital stays and less pain following surgery, with better results in terms of symptom reduction and restoration of esophageal function.

Esophagectomy: Esophagectomy may be necessary in end-stage achalasia patients with significant esophageal dilatation, sigmoid-like oesophagus, or esophageal cancer in order to treat the underlying disease and stop additional problems. Surgical alternatives include esophagectomy with or without reconstruction, depending on the disease stage and treatment objectives of each patient.

Endoscopic Anti-Reflux Procedures: Patients with achalasia frequently have concurrent gastroesophageal reflux disease (GERD). To prevent postoperative reflux and improve long-term outcomes, endoscopic anti-reflux procedures like fundoplication may be performed concurrently with myotomy for those patients who have significant reflux symptoms or documented esophagitis.

The long-term results of surgical procedures for achalasia have shown promise in terms of improved esophageal function, patient satisfaction, and symptom reduction. High success rates for esophageal emptying and symptom alleviation have been documented in studies; also, there is a low risk of procedure-related side effects and long-lasting effectiveness. Moreover, the development of minimally invasive procedures has improved the overall effectiveness of surgical treatments for achalasia by lowering postoperative morbidity and speeding recovery.

Thorough preoperative evaluation, individualised perioperative care, and careful patient selection are essential for the effective application of surgical methods in the therapy of achalasia. In order to identify the best surgical intervention and maximise postoperative outcomes, factors including the patient's age, comorbidities, esophageal function, and disease stage are crucial. Furthermore, to ensure the best outcomes for patients undergoing surgical care for achalasia, multidisciplinary teamwork between gastroenterologists, surgeons, anesthesiologists, and nutritionists is essential in providing thorough preoperative optimization and postoperative support.

Finally, taking surgical options into account while managing achalasia is an essential part of providing a full range of patient care, especially when endoscopic therapies may not be sufficient or when advanced disease stages or consequences need definitive surgery. Healthcare professionals must have a thorough understanding of the indications, surgical intervention types, expected outcomes, and perioperative considerations in order to help patients make informed decisions and carry out individualised treatment plans that maximise symptomatic relief, esophageal function, and quality of life in people with achalasia.

Botox Injections: A Temporary Relief

When it comes to the treatment of achalasia, Botox injections are an additional therapeutic option for patients who might not be a good fit for or have not responded well to conventional procedures like surgical myotomy or pneumatic dilatation. This chapter explores the advantages, restrictions, and procedural nuances of using Botox injections to treat the symptoms of achalasia.

In order to temporarily paralyse the sphincter muscle, botulinum toxin is directly injected into the lower esophageal sphincter (LES) during a botox injection, also known as a botulinum toxin injection. By reducing the functional obstruction at the LES, this neuromuscular blockade seeks to improve esophageal emptying and lessen dysphagia in achalasia patients.

Botox injections are essential for managing achalasia because they can temporarily interfere with the faulty function of the sphincter, relieving symptoms and promoting better esophageal transit. For certain patients, particularly those who are contraindicated to other therapies or who require a bridge therapy while they await definitive interventions, Botox injections provide a transient yet valuable therapeutic option, in contrast to permanent interventions like dilatation or myotomy.

Botulinum toxin was first used to treat blepharospasm and strabismus, which led to its introduction as a neuromuscular blocking agent with a variety of clinical uses. This use is where the toxin's use in medical therapy begins. The armamentarium of therapeutic options accessible to individuals with this difficult esophageal motility problem has increased with the development of Botox injections as a viable therapy technique for achalasia.

In addition to the range of endoscopic and surgical treatments available for achalasia, Botox injections are a crucial part of the multidisciplinary approach to managing this problem. Botox injections are a beneficial adjuvant in the comprehensive management of patients with achalasia due to their temporary nature and particular indications. They address distinct clinical circumstances and optimise treatment outcomes.

Botox injections are used for achalasia in patients who are not candidates for traditional therapies, such as high surgical risk patients or those with concurrent medical conditions that prohibit invasive operations. In situations when definitive procedures are planned for a later time, Botox injections can also be used as a bridge therapy to provide temporary symptom relief and improve nutritional status while waiting for permanent answers.

Regarding the long-term durability and efficacy of Botox injections in the management of achalasia, there is a prevalent misperception. It is important to understand that Botox injections only provide short-term comfort and may require additional treatment because of their reversible effect. As a result, patients and medical professionals need to understand that the symptomatic relief brought on by Botox injections is temporary and that further monitoring and treatment planning are necessary.

Injections of Botox offer several advantages in the treatment of achalasia, especially in certain clinical situations where a transient therapeutic strategy is necessary. These benefits include being minimally invasive, being appropriate for individuals who are contraindicated for other procedures, and having the potential to serve as a bridge therapy in some situations.

Because Botox injections are a minimally invasive technique, they are a popular choice for patients who are contraindicated for or uncomfortable with more invasive endoscopic or surgical procedures. For those with achalasia, the peroral administration of Botox injections through endoscopy is a well-tolerated intervention because it involves little discomfort during the procedure and quick recovery thereafter.

The temporising effect of Botox injections may be beneficial for patients with significant comorbidities or those who are considered high surgical risk due to underlying medical conditions, as it offers symptomatic relief without exposing them to the possible risks associated with more invasive interventions.

When more permanent procedures like surgical myotomy or pneumatic dilatation are planned for a later date, Botox injections act as a bridge therapy to reduce dysphagia and enhance nutritional status during this time. While waiting for long-term remedies, this temporising impact is very helpful in improving patient well-being and optimising the overall care of achalasia.

Even if Botox injections have significant advantages in some therapeutic situations, it's important to understand their drawbacks and take particular factors into account when implementing them into the achalasia treatment plan.

Botox injections have a temporary therapeutic effect that requires periodic re-administration since the neuromuscular blockage caused by the toxin can be reversed. As a result, patients receiving Botox injections should be made aware that the symptomatic relief they experience is only momentary and that they may require follow-up appointments and maybe more injections.

In patients with underlying esophageal dysmotility and impaired esophageal clearance, in particular, Botox injections may aggravate symptoms of gastroesophageal reflux by temporarily paralysing the lower esophageal sphincter. Consequently, when choosing patients for Botox injections, thorough evaluation of the risk-benefit profile is essential, particularly when coexisting gastric reflux illness is present (GERD).

A thorough evaluation of each patient's unique clinical features, such as esophageal function, comorbidities, and treatment objectives, is necessary for the wise selection of patients for Botox injections in the management of achalasia. In addition, careful monitoring and treatment planning are crucial parts of the continuity of care for patients receiving Botox injections, guaranteeing prompt reassessment and possible transfer to permanent therapies as necessary.

When it comes to managing achalasia, the procedural components of giving Botox injections involve particular methods and factors to maximise the intervention's effectiveness and safety.

Botox injections are usually given intraperitoneally (IV) under endoscopic supervision, which enables accurate localization and administration into the lower eyelid (LES). Endoscopic visualisation reduces the possibility of an unintentional puncture or injury during the treatment and guarantees precise injection placement.

Botox injection dose and placement are customised based on each patient's unique LES features and esophageal motility patterns, taking into account both the intended outcome and preventing excessive toxin diffusion outside of the targeted sphincter region.

After receiving a Botox injection, patients are closely watched for any post-procedural symptoms and have follow-up appointments set up to determine whether further injections are necessary and how long the symptomatic relief lasts. By using an organised method, the therapeutic value of Botox injections will be maximised, and the patient's clinical reaction will inform future treatment decisions.

To sum up, Botox injections are a useful addition to the overall treatment of achalasia, providing some patients with a transient but effective therapeutic choice. The multifaceted approach to achalasia care is highlighted by their position as a minimally invasive, temporising intervention in various clinical circumstances, such as patients who are awaiting definitive therapies or who are contraindicated to traditional treatments. Healthcare professionals can optimise the therapy protocol for achalasia, addressing a variety of clinical circumstances and improving patient outcomes in this difficult esophageal motility disorder, by carefully considering the advantages, drawbacks, and procedural nuances of Botox injections.

The Role of Diet in Managing Symptoms

The main objectives of dietary management for those with achalasia are to reduce symptoms and enhance general quality of life for those who suffer from this difficult esophageal motility condition. Patients can improve their nutritional status and overall well-being by reducing the effects of dysphagia, regurgitation, and related discomfort through dietary modifications and mealtime practises.

People should be well informed on achalasia and how it affects esophageal function before starting any dietary changes for the management of the condition. Furthermore, it's crucial to speak with a licenced healthcare professional, such as a registered dietitian or gastroenterologist, to customise dietary advice to each patient's unique requirements and tolerances.

In order to maximise esophageal transit and reduce symptoms, dietary management of achalasia involves a multifaceted approach that integrates changes in food texture, meal frequency, and eating patterns. The main tactics include addressing potential dietary triggers, creating a supportive eating environment, and modifying meal size and consistency to promote safe swallowing.

Modifying the texture of food is essential for compensating for the reduced esophageal clearance that is a hallmark of achalasia. Foods that are soft, moist, and readily swallowed are recommended in order to reduce the possibility of aspiration and obstruction. Foods that have had their texture altered include creamy soups, pureed veggies, mashed fruits, and tender meats. It helps to prevent dysphagia and encourage comfortable swallowing to emphasise foods that need little chewing and pass easily down the oesophagus.

Meals that are divided into smaller, more frequent portions can improve dietary intake and lessen the strain on the oesophagus. Eating fewer meals at a time promotes more effective digestion and absorption by lowering the risk of esophageal stasis and regurgitation.

Furthermore, distributing meals throughout the day and allowing enough time between meals helps food pass slowly down the oesophagus, which reduces achalasia symptoms.

Drinking lots of liquids together with your meals can help the food travel down your oesophagus and support the propulsion of boluses. Soups, stews, and smoothies are examples of foods high in fluid content that help lubricate food particles in the stomach and facilitate esophageal passage, which reduces dysphagia and improves overall meal tolerance. However, to avoid aggravating symptoms like reflux and discomfort, careful thought should be given to the temperature and volume of beverages.

Effective dietary therapy of achalasia requires the identification and avoidance of dietary triggers that increase symptoms of the condition. Carbonated drinks, spicy meals, citrus or acidic fruits, and foods high in fat or fibre are examples of common triggers. People can reduce their chance of experiencing discomfort, regurgitation, and esophageal spasm by consuming less of these possible irritants. This will increase their ability to tolerate meals and manage their symptoms.

Changes in posture and eating habits can have a big impact on how easy it is to swallow and lessen the chance that symptoms will get worse. Techniques include eating slowly, chewing food well, and taking little bits help break down solid food particles and make it easier for food to pass down the oesophagus safely. Additionally, by keeping your posture straight during and after meals, you can minimise discomfort and optimise esophageal transit by preventing reflux and regurgitation.

- People who have achalasia should always stay well hydrated during the day since drinking enough fluids helps with esophageal clearance and bolus propulsion.

- To make sure that vital macro- and micronutrient requirements are satisfied, careful consideration should be given to the nutritional sufficiency of the diet when making dietary modifications.

- Incorporating meals high in fibre, like cooked veggies and soft fruits, can help encourage regular bowel movements and reduce constipation, which is a typical issue among patients with achalasia.

Dietary changes that effectively manage the symptoms of achalasia can be verified by measuring improvements in meal tolerance, subjective symptom improvement, and reduced occurrences of regurgitation and dysphagia. Maintaining regular contact with a dietician or healthcare professional can help with tracking dietary changes and how they affect symptom management.

When dietary changes by themselves are insufficient to relieve symptoms, further measures like myotomy, pneumatic dilatation, or medication management can be necessary. Working together with medical professionals is crucial to overcoming any obstacles in managing symptoms and investigating other forms of treatment.

To sum up, the deliberate application of dietary adjustments is a fundamental component of the all-encompassing treatment of achalasia, providing people with the chance to take charge of their symptoms and enhance their nutritional status. Healthcare professionals can help patients manage achalasia with more resilience and confidence by customising dietary recommendations to meet their individual needs and dietary restrictions. This will ultimately improve the patients' quality of life despite this complex esophageal motility disorder.

Emerging Therapies: Future of Achalasia Treatment

Achalasia is a challenging esophageal motility disorder characterized by impaired relaxation of the lower esophageal sphincter and absent peristalsis in the esophageal body, leading to dysphagia, regurgitation, chest pain, and weight loss. Traditional treatment approaches including pneumatic dilation, surgical myotomy, and botulinum toxin injection have demonstrated efficacy in symptom management. However, emerging therapies and investigational treatments are poised to revolutionize the landscape of achalasia management, offering novel avenues for improving esophageal function and enhancing patient outcomes. This section will explore the current status and future potential of these innovative approaches, shedding light on their promise in reshaping the management of achalasia.

:The emergence of novel therapies and investigational treatments presents a paradigm shift in the management of achalasia, offering unprecedented opportunities for targeted symptom relief and functional restoration. These advancements have the potential to redefine the standard of care for achalasia, addressing unmet needs and enhancing the overall quality of life for individuals living with this complex esophageal disorder.

:One of the most promising emerging therapies for achalasia is peroral endoscopic myotomy (POEM), a minimally invasive procedure that involves creating a submucosal tunnel in the esophagus and performing a selective myotomy of the inner circular muscle fibers of the lower esophageal sphincter. Several studies have demonstrated the efficacy of POEM in achieving sustained symptomatic relief and improving esophageal function in patients with achalasia. Notably, POEM has been shown to offer comparable or even superior outcomes to traditional treatment modalities, with lower complication rates and shorter hospital stays.

The rationale behind POEM lies in its ability to achieve a tailored myotomy of the lower esophageal sphincter, addressing the underlying pathophysiology of achalasia while minimizing trauma to the esophageal mucosa. By leveraging advanced endoscopic techniques, POEM enables precise dissection and myotomy, resulting in durable symptom control and functional improvement. Furthermore, the minimally invasive nature of POEM translates to reduced postoperative pain, faster recovery, and improved patient satisfaction, underscoring its potential as a transformative intervention in achalasia management.

:While POEM has garnered significant attention as a promising alternative to traditional surgical interventions for achalasia, concerns have been raised regarding its long-term durability and the potential for gastroesophageal reflux disease (GERD) post-procedure. Some studies have reported an increased incidence of post-POEM reflux, raising questions about the necessity for concomitant antireflux measures and long-term surveillance for reflux-related complications. Additionally, the learning curve associated with mastering the technical intricacies of POEM may pose challenges in ensuring consistent and reproducible outcomes across different centers and practitioners.

:Despite the apprehensions surrounding post-POEM reflux, recent evidence suggests that meticulous patient selection, tailored myotomy length, and adjunctive antireflux strategies can mitigate the risk of GERD following POEM. Studies have highlighted the importance of pre-procedural evaluation of esophageal acid exposure and esophageal motility patterns to identify patients at higher risk for post-POEM reflux, facilitating personalized management strategies. Moreover, ongoing advancements in endoscopic imaging and functional testing hold promise for refining the selection criteria and optimizing outcomes with POEM, addressing the concerns related to long-term efficacy and reflux control.

:In addition to POEM, emerging endoscopic therapies such as peroral endoscopic fundoplication (PEF) and endoscopic pyloromyotomy (EP) have emerged as potential adjuncts to achalasia management. PEF offers a minimally invasive approach to reinforce the antireflux barrier following myotomy, addressing the concerns of post-procedural reflux and enhancing the overall efficacy of POEM. Similarly, EP targets concomitant gastroparesis or pyloric dysfunction, addressing the functional disturbances beyond the esophagus that can contribute to persistent symptoms in achalasia. These complementary endoscopic interventions hold promise in optimizing the comprehensive management of achalasia and addressing the multifaceted nature of the disease.

:The advent of novel therapies and investigational treatments in the management of achalasia represents a transformative juncture in addressing the unmet needs of individuals living with this complex esophageal disorder. While challenges and uncertainties persist, the evidence supporting the efficacy and safety of emerging interventions such as POEM, PEF, and EP underscores their potential to redefine the standard of care for achalasia, offering tailored and minimally invasive alternatives to traditional surgical approaches. As ongoing research continues to unravel the intricacies of these innovative therapies, their integration into the clinical armamentarium holds the promise of reshaping the landscape of achalasia management, ultimately improving patient outcomes and quality of life.

Choosing the Right Treatment: A Personalized Approach

Due to compromised lower esophageal sphincter relaxation and missing esophageal peristalsis, achalasia, a rare esophageal motility condition, frequently causes dysphagia, regurgitation, chest discomfort, and weight loss. Although symptomatic alleviation has been achieved with the traditional therapeutic procedures of pneumatic dilatation, surgical myotomy, and botulinum toxin injection, new research points to the possibility of revolutionary improvements in the field of achalasia management. The purpose of this section is to assist patients in choosing the best treatment option possible given their unique needs and circumstances.

The lack of a technique that works for everyone in managing achalasia is one of the main problems. Personalized treatment plans are necessary since every patient has a different clinical presentation, set of comorbidities, and set of therapeutic objectives. The lack of a defined strategy to choose the best course of action can lead to less than ideal results and a prolonged burden of symptoms for patients.

Ignoring the reality that achalasia treatment is customised can result in treatment failure, symptom recurrence, and the requirement for further therapies. Furthermore, ignoring patient-specific considerations during the decision-making process may lead to needless procedural difficulties and resource consumption.

A individualised approach that takes into account the patient's preferences, the severity of the condition, anatomical concerns, and potential post-treatment problems is crucial to address the multidimensional character of achalasia and enhance treatment outcomes. The total efficacy and patient satisfaction can be maximised by customising the treatment plan to each patient's specific situation.

A thorough evaluation of the patient's clinical profile, including symptom severity, esophageal architecture, concomitant diseases, and therapeutic preferences, is necessary before implementing a tailored approach. The patient's general state of health, any potential contraindications to particular therapies, and the accessibility of specialised facilities offering cutting-edge treatment methods should all be taken into account during this examination.

The advantages of individualised treatment plans for achalasia management have been emphasised by numerous research. Better treatment outcomes and increased quality of life have been documented when the treatment plan is customised to the unique patient's age, symptom duration, and esophageal motility patterns. Making educated decisions and maximising patient satisfaction can be facilitated by predictive modelling that takes into account patient-specific characteristics to offer insights into the likelihood of success for different treatment approaches.

Although a customised strategy offers specialised solutions for managing achalasia, it's critical to recognise that there are other available therapeutic options. These could involve investigating minimally invasive surgical procedures, developing complementing pharmaceutical therapy, or developing innovative endoscopic interventions. Patients and healthcare providers can make well-informed therapy decisions by weighing the relative efficacy, safety profiles, and long-term results of different options.

As precision medicine progresses and the diversity of achalasia is increasingly acknowledged, the paradigm for managing the condition is changing to one that is more patient-centered and individualised. It is possible to determine the best course of action for each patient by combining their preferences, the features of their illness, and evidence-based interventions. This approach ultimately improves patient happiness and optimises therapeutic outcomes.

Meal Planning and Preparation: Strategies for Success

Planning and preparing meals is a crucial part of controlling achalasia because it enables people to modify their eating patterns to meet the demands of the illness. We will explore the complexities of meal planning and preparation for patients with Achalasia in this chapter, offering a thorough manual to assist people in confidently and easily navigating their particular dietary requirements.

:1. Selecting Achalasia-Friendly Foods
2. Texture Modification Techniques
3. Portion Control and Timing
4. Creating a Supportive Meal Environment
5. Implementing Adaptive Eating Strategies

:1. Selecting Achalasia-Friendly Foods

The selection of Achalasia-In order to ensure that people with Achalasia can eat their meals safely and pleasantly, friendly foods are essential. These foods ought to be simple to eat, easily accepted, and unlikely to cause symptoms like regurgitation or dysphagia.

Achalasia-Soft, moist, and easily digested foods like pureed fruits, cooked vegetables, and tender meats are examples of friendly foods. In addition, despite possible difficulties with swallowing and digestion, people can still satisfy their nutritional needs by including high-protein foods and nutrient-dense options.

Studies have demonstrated the advantages of a soft diet for those with Achalasia, stressing the significance of choosing meals that are easy on the oesophagus and allow for easy passage into the stomach. Testimonials from people who have Achalasia also highlight the benefits of customised meal choices for their general health and symptom management.

To find options that are easy to eat and pleasurable, it's useful to experiment with different textures, flavours, and cooking techniques when choosing foods that are suitable for Achalasia. Choosing foods based on personal preferences and dietary needs can be further optimised by working with a nutritionist or dietitian.

The basis for effective meal planning and preparation is the thoughtful selection of foods that are suitable for Achalasia. Soft, moist, and nutrient-dense foods are the ones that people should prioritise in order to build a framework that will help them efficiently manage their nutritional demands.

2. Texture Modification Techniques

Overview:

Techniques for texturizing food include changing its texture and consistency to make it easier for those with Achalasia to consume. These methods are intended to make swallowing easier and reduce the possibility of food being stuck in the oesophagus.

To achieve a smoother and more consistent texture, solid foods might be blended, pureed, or mashed. These are common texture modification procedures. Furthermore, adding moisture-rich components and thickening liquids can improve the modified foods' overall swallowability and palatability, making them simpler for patients with Achalasia to tolerate.

Research on patients with Achalasia has shown that texture modification is beneficial in enhancing swallowing function and lowering the frequency of dysphagia-related problems. Testimonials from people who have used texture modification techniques highlight the benefits even more for their overall eating experience and treatment of symptoms.

In order to attain the best consistency and swallowability, practical texture modification techniques need experimenting with different food textures and investigating different preparation processes. For added convenience, the texture alteration process can be streamlined by using specialty kitchen gear and appliances like food processors and blenders. Texture modification techniques provide a flexible way to modify food textures and consistency to meet the specific requirements of people with Achalasia. Through the application of these procedures, people might broaden their culinary horizons and relish a variety of altered delicacies that are both gratifying and secure to eat.

3. Portion Control and Timing

For people with achalasia, portion control and timing are very important since they can help control symptoms including dysphagia, regurgitation, and discomfort during and after meals. People can maximise their nutritional intake and reduce their chance of experiencing symptoms by eating at the right times and in the right portions.

Eating smaller, more frequent meals helps minimise the amount of food that enters the oesophagus at any one moment, which lowers the risk of reflux and blockage. Additionally, esophageal sphincter pressure can be reduced and easier food passage into the stomach can be encouraged by spacing out meals and giving the stomach enough time to digest.

Clinical studies have demonstrated the advantages of portion control and meal scheduling in the management of Achalasia symptoms, emphasising the beneficial effects on the ability to swallow, the intensity of symptoms, and general quality of life. Testimonials from those who have used these techniques attest to their further efficacy in fostering relaxation and digestive health.

In order to achieve optimal digestion and reduce symptoms, it is important to plan and prepare smaller, nutrient-dense meals throughout the day and to provide enough time between them. This is known as portion control and timing. Furthermore, mindful eating techniques like chewing well and eating slowly can help with quantity control and meal scheduling. Individuals diagnosed with Achalasia can effectively manage their dietary problems and achieve maximum digestion and comfort by adopting portion management and strategically timing their meals. By customising each meal to their specific needs and tastes, these strategies enable people to confidently manage their meal routines.

4. Creating a Supportive Meal Environment

For people with Achalasia, it is crucial to create a supportive dining environment because it creates a welcoming and accommodative atmosphere that encourages comfort, enjoyment, and relaxation during meals. People can limit potential triggers for symptoms and improve their overall dining experience by improving the meal setting.

Creating a peaceful, stress-free setting, minimising distractions, and promoting mindful eating and comfortable swallowing are all components of supportive meal environments. For those who have Achalasia, choosing suitable seating arrangements and mealtime settings can also improve the whole dining experience.

Research in psychology has demonstrated how the setting of a meal affects eating habits and digestive comfort. It has also highlighted how important a supportive environment is for encouraging relaxation, lowering anxiety, and maximising meal satisfaction. Testimonials from people who have Achalasia also highlight the benefits of a mealtime atmosphere that is supportive for managing symptoms and general well-being.

Incorporating relaxing aspects like soft lighting and quiet music, designating specific meal places free from distractions, and practising relaxation techniques before and during meals to generate a sense of ease and comfort are all useful tactics for creating a supportive dining environment. Furthermore, having uplifting interactions and dialogues during meals might improve the whole dining experience. People can create an eating environment that supports their specific requirements and encourages enjoyment and relaxation during meals by making the establishment of a supportive meal environment a priority. These factors enable people to make the most out of their mealtime experiences and reduce any tensions that can interfere with their ability to eat peacefully.

5. Implementing Adaptive Eating Strategies

Adaptive eating strategies are a collection of methods and approaches intended to help people with Achalasia eat comfortably and effectively. By addressing particular issues with swallowing, digestion, and food enjoyment, these tactics hope to improve the overall dining experience for those with Achalasia.

To maximise food breakdown and swallowability, common adaptive eating tactics include using smaller utensils, taking smaller bits, and using the proper chewing techniques. Achalasia sufferers can also benefit from the ease and comfort of eating by combining supportive postures and attentive breathing techniques.

The usefulness of adaptive eating techniques in encouraging meal consumption, lowering the incidence of symptoms, and improving overall eating satisfaction for people with Achalasia has been demonstrated by clinical research. Individuals who have adopted adaptive eating practises have provided testimonials that emphasise the beneficial effects on their mealtime experiences and management of symptoms.

In order to maximise mealtime comfort and efficiency, adaptive eating tactics can be practically implemented by including small utensils, practising attentive chewing and swallowing procedures, and experimenting with supportive postures. Furthermore, mindful breathing techniques and relaxation methods might enhance adaptive eating tactics by encouraging a feeling of comfort and wellbeing throughout meals. Through the integration of adaptive eating methods into their mealtime routines, people with Achalasia can more confidently and easily handle their dietary issues. By enabling people to consume meals with awareness and flexibility, these tactics guarantee that every meal is customised to the individual's requirements and tastes.

Conclusion:

Achalasia patients have specific dietary demands and preparation requirements, therefore meal planning and preparation must take careful consideration, strategic methods, and adaptive strategies into account. People can create a comforting and fulfilling dining experience that enhances comfort, contentment, and general well-being by adopting the previously described tactics into their mealtime routines. People can confidently and masterfully navigate their dietary journey, optimising their mealtime experiences and improving their overall quality of life, by carefully choosing Achalasia-friendly foods, modifying their texture, controlling portion sizes and timing, creating a supportive meal environment, and putting adaptive eating strategies into practise.

Eating Techniques: Minimizing Discomfort

This section's main objective is to provide people with Achalasia with practical eating strategies that help reduce their discomfort during meals, improving their entire dining experience and encouraging improved symptom management.

It is crucial for people to have a fundamental awareness of their unique Achalasia symptoms and triggers before diving into the eating practises. For the recommended strategies to be effectively implemented, it is also essential to have access to soft, moist, and readily digestible foods, as well as appropriate utensils and mealtime settings.

The eating strategies covered in this part are meant to help with the difficulties related to Achalasia, like regurgitation and dysphagia, by encouraging efficient and comfortable meal ingestion. These methods address posture, pacing, and chewing, among other areas of the eating process, in an effort to reduce discomfort and maximise the dining experience for those with Achalasia.

1. Chewing Techniques for Achalasia Management

For people with achalasia, safe and easy swallowing is greatly aided by effective chewing methods. People who chew their food properly can help break it down into smaller, easier-to-digest pieces, which lowers the chance of food impaction and pain when swallowing.

Chewing is an essential part of the early phases of digestion because it makes food mechanically break down into a bolus that passes smoothly down the oesophagus. A slow and thorough chewing technique can help ensure that food is sufficiently prepared for swallowing in those with Achalasia, reducing the strain on the esophageal sphincter and facilitating a smoother passage into the stomach.

Research has shown how crucial good chewing habits are for maximising swallowing efficiency and lowering the frequency of dysphagia-related problems in Achalasia patients. Testimonials from people who have adopted particular chewing techniques emphasise the beneficial effects on their dining experiences and symptom management even more.

Effective chewing strategies can be practically used by chewing mindfully, taking smaller, more deliberate bites, and making sure that each bite is fully masticated before swallowing. They can also be made even more effective by adding supportive postures and making sure you give yourself enough time to chew.

2. Pacing Strategies for Comfortable Meal Consumption

In order to decrease discomfort and encourage safe swallowing, pacing measures are crucial for people with Achalasia to manage their meal consumption successfully. They help regulate the speed and rhythm of eating. People can enhance their ability to chew, swallow, and breathe during meals by using the right pacing strategies.

Eating with purpose and control requires the use of spacing techniques, which include chewing food well, taking regular rests between bites, and giving the food enough time to pass easily down the oesophagus. These tactics are designed to reduce the possibility of regurgitation and discomfort during and after meals, as well as to stop food from building up in the oesophagus.

The advantages of pacing techniques in encouraging efficient and comfortable meal consumption for people with Achalasia have been highlighted in clinical literature, with particular attention to the beneficial effects on swallowing coordination and general mealtime pleasure. Testimonials from people who have adopted pacing techniques provide as additional evidence of how successful these tactics are at reducing discomfort and fostering digestive health.

Setting a steady and comfortable eating pace, pausing frequently to check on swallowing comfort, and paying attention to the timing of chewing, swallowing, and breathing are all examples of how pacing techniques can be put into practise. In addition, pacing tactics can be further enhanced by establishing a meal environment that supports leisurely and unhurried feeding.

- Guidelines for Efficient Chewing and Pacing: - Engage in mindful eating by paying attention to the flavour, texture, and scent of every bite.

- To promote smaller bites and improve chewing efficiency, use smaller silverware or utensils.

To lessen discomfort and increase mealtime happiness, emphasis taking your time when eating and avoid hurrying through meals.

Cautionary Notes Regarding Possible Difficulties: - People who are used to fast or rushed eating habits may find it difficult at first to get used to new chewing and pacing methods.

- The excessive extension of meal duration resulting from the overzealous application of pacing tactics may cause a decline in meal enjoyment and satiety.

The effectiveness of the chewing and pacing procedures can be confirmed by measuring improvements in overall mealtime pleasure, the occurrence of symptoms related to dysphagia being less frequent, and the comfort of meals. By recording their experiences in a food diary or notebook, people can track their development and spot any trends or advancements in their comfort level when eating.

If people find it difficult to adjust to the recommended chewing and pacing methods, they should consult a skilled nutritionist or healthcare provider. They can offer individualised help and customised advice to address particular issues or implementation barriers. Furthermore, practising mindful eating and progressively incorporating the methods into regular mealtime routines can help get beyond early obstacles and maximise the benefits of the approaches.

In summary, the efficient application of chewing and pacing strategies is essential to reducing discomfort and fostering the best possible mealtime experiences for people with Achalasia. Individuals can improve their mealtime happiness, facilitate safe and comfortable swallowing, and eventually become proficient in managing their dietary issues connected to Achalasia by adopting intentional and thoughtful approaches to chewing and pacing.

The Impact of Exercise on Achalasia

The topic of exercise's effects on Achalasia is complex and includes both possible advantages and disadvantages of physical activity for those who have this esophageal motility condition. Swallowing and digesting are severely hampered by achalasia, an uncommon disorder marked by decreased esophageal peristalsis and insufficient relaxation of the lower esophageal sphincter. Exercise, on the other hand, encompasses a wide variety of physical activities that can have a variety of consequences on the body, such as changes in the musculoskeletal system, metabolism, and cardiovascular system.

The purpose of comparing the effects of exercise and Achalasia is to clarify how physical activity may help manage the symptoms of Achalasia, treat related comorbidities, and improve the general health of those who are affected. This investigation attempts to contribute to a more thorough understanding of the management of Achalasia by shedding light on the complex interaction between physical activity and esophageal motility problems by analysing the confluence of exercise and Achalasia.

It is crucial to take into account the possible physiological, psychological, and symptomatic impacts of various forms of physical activity when assessing the influence of exercise on Achalasia. The quality of life, symptom severity, esophageal function, and the management of comorbid illnesses like depression and anxiety that are frequently linked to Achalasia are among the benchmarks used for comparison.

Exercise that is customised for each patient's situation may help those with Achalasia have better digestive and esophageal motility. Frequent exercise can improve general physical health, cardiovascular fitness, and muscular tone, all of which can indirectly boost esophageal function and strengthen the body's ability to adapt to problems associated with Achalasia. Furthermore, certain workouts that focus on respiratory capacity, postural alignment, and relaxation techniques may directly help to reduce esophageal discomfort and promote comfort during meals and daily activities.

On the other hand, several types of exercise—especially those that require vigorous physical effort, sudden posture adjustments, or valsalva maneuvers—may make symptoms of dysphagia and regurgitation worse in people with Achalasia. Excessive exercise has the potential to cause discomfort during or after physical activity, raise intra-abdominal pressure, and cause esophageal spasms. Achalasia sufferers may also have anxiety associated with the worry that they would aspirate or impaction food while exercising, which makes it more difficult for them to participate in several forms of physical activity.

Visual aids can improve the clarity and understanding of the contrasts and comparisons offered. Examples of these are diagrams that show the possible effects of various training modalities on esophageal function and symptom severity. Furthermore, graphical depictions of suggested workouts and safety measures for people with Achalasia might offer helpful advice for integrating exercise into everyday routines while lowering hazards.

When exercise and Achalasia are compared, it becomes clear that how physical activity affects esophageal function and symptom management depends on the kind, level, and tolerance of the individual to exercise. It is crucial to have a sophisticated awareness of the possible advantages and disadvantages of various physical activities in order to customise exercise regimens to the particular requirements and limitations of people with Achalasia. Furthermore, the incorporation of specific workouts and relaxation methods can provide beneficial supplementary assistance in managing the complex issues presented by Achalasia, which include both physiological and psychological aspects.

The incorporation of exercise as an adjunctive strategy for managing Achalasia is consistent with the patient-centered care model and customised treatment plans in the context of modern healthcare and wellness initiatives. Given that exercise has the potential to improve esophageal function and overall well-being in people with Achalasia, healthcare professionals and the affected individuals can work together to develop customised exercise programmes that support symptom relief, functional ability, and psychological fortitude in the face of long-term health issues.

In summary, the benefits of exercise on Achalasia require a more nuanced knowledge of the complex interactions between physical activity and abnormalities of the esophageal motility than a simple binary assessment of helpful or negative effects. Through a critical evaluation of the potential benefits and drawbacks of exercise in the context of Achalasia, both individuals and medical professionals can develop customised and knowledgeable strategies for incorporating physical activity as an auxiliary element of overall Achalasia management.

Stress Management and Achalasia

Achalasia and stress have a complex relationship that raises a lot of questions about esophageal motility issues. Psychological and emotional stressors can have a significant impact on achalasia, a condition marked by impaired esophageal peristalsis and sphincter dysfunction. The complex interaction that exists between stress and symptoms of Achalasia calls for a thorough investigation to clarify the possible consequences for symptom exacerbation and disease management. Comprehending this relationship is essential to developing comprehensive strategies for the treatment of Achalasia that take into account both the physiological and psychological aspects.

The main concern here is how stress affects the symptoms of Achalasia and how psychological worry may exacerbate esophageal dysfunction. Swallowing difficulties, regurgitation, and discomfort during meals are common issues for people with achalasia, and these issues can be made worse by stress and anxiety. Because of this, the complex nature of the problem demands careful thought in order to lessen any potential negative consequences on the management of achalasia.

Untreated stress and Achalasia symptoms can lead to increased symptom intensity, worse quality of life, and increased psychological distress for those affected by this esophageal motility condition. Unmanaged stress in the context of Achalasia can have negative effects on emotional health and coping mechanisms in addition to the physical symptoms of the illness. Furthermore, prolonged symptom load and subpar treatment outcomes may result from the persistence of unrelenting stress, which could undermine the effectiveness of traditional Achalasia treatments and interventions.

The complex association between stress and Achalasia calls for the inclusion of psychological therapies and stress-reduction approaches as a critical strategy to improve general well-being and disease management. Through the application of evidence-based stress management techniques, people with Achalasia may be able to reduce the negative effects of stress on their symptoms, develop psychological fortitude, and enhance their ability to manage the difficulties this long-term illness presents.

The application of stress management strategies for people with Achalasia requires a customised strategy that recognises the particular requirements and constraints that this patient population possesses. To improve psychological well-being and coping abilities, cognitive-behavioral therapy, mindfulness-based interventions, relaxation techniques, and stress-reduction tactics can be incorporated into the all-encompassing care of people with Achalasia. In addition, it is imperative that mental health specialists and healthcare practitioners work together to develop customised stress management programmes that meet the unique needs of people with Achalasia.

Research indicates that implementing stress-reduction strategies in the treatment of long-term medical problems can result in positive results such as reduced symptom severity, better quality of life, and increased psychological well-being. Based on the results of similar conditions, people with Achalasia may benefit from stress management interventions in the following ways: they may experience fewer episodes of exacerbation of symptoms, better adherence to treatment, and an overall increase in resilience to the difficulties this complex esophageal disorder presents.

The utilisation of complementary approaches, like biofeedback, meditation, and supportive counselling, may expand the range of strategies available for addressing the psychological aspects of Achalasia, even though stress management techniques remain a crucial intervention for reducing the impact of stress on the condition. The assessment of substitute approaches recognises the complex character of stress and its consequences for managing Achalasia, so facilitating a thorough framework for advancing the overall health of impacted individuals.

In summary, the complex relationship between stress and Achalasia emphasises how important it is to incorporate evidence-based stress management strategies into the all-encompassing care of patients suffering from this esophageal motility condition. Acknowledging the possible effects of unchecked stress on symptoms of Achalasia and psychological health, medical professionals and patients alike can work together to investigate customised stress-reduction techniques that build resilience, improve coping mechanisms, and maximise the treatment of this intricate chronic illness.

Navigating Social Situations With Achalasia

This chapter's main goal is to provide people with Achalasia with useful coping mechanisms for social circumstances, especially when it comes to going out to eat and attending activities. The goal is to enable readers to participate in social events with ease and confidence, improving their overall quality of life, by offering thorough information on managing the emotional and social obstacles related to Achalasia.

To achieve the goal of adeptly navigating social situations with Achalasia, individuals may benefit from possessing the following prerequisites:

- A basic comprehension of the symptoms of Achalasia and how they affect day-to-day activities.

- Knowledge of dietary adjustments and eating methods specific to the treatment of achalasia.

- a readiness to speak up for their demands through proactive engagement with peers, restaurant employees, and event organisers.

- Availability of suitable resources to support comfortable meal experiences, such as specially designed seating arrangements or adaptive eating utensils.

Navigating social situations with Achalasia involves a multi-faceted approach encompassing proactive communication, strategic meal planning, and the cultivation of coping mechanisms to address potential challenges. The process can be delineated into the following key steps:

1. Preparing for social events by assessing the environment and potential accommodations.

2. Communicating effectively with peers, hosts, and restaurant staff to convey specific dietary and seating requirements.

3. Implementing practical strategies for managing symptoms and discomfort during social gatherings.

4. Cultivating a proactive mindset and building resilience to mitigate the impact of social challenges on emotional well-being.

- Familiarize yourself with the venue: Examine the venue's accessibility, seating configurations, and food options before going to a social event or dining out. Planning ahead for possible obstacles or modifications will help you manage the event more skillfully.

- Plan your meal choices: Examine the menu selections and pay attention to the dishes' textures, temperatures, and serving sizes. Choose lighter, more easily digested foods and ask if any menu items may be changed or customised to meet your specific dietary requirements.

- Identify potential accommodations: When feasible, talk with the event organisers or the restaurant staff to make specific requests for seating arrangements or modifications, such as elevated seats, cushions for support, or easy access to the facilities.

- Advocate for your needs: Make sure you are clear and forceful when communicating your dietary needs and preferred seating arrangements to the host or restaurant personnel before the event. Describe your illness, any restrictions it may have, and any modifications that may improve your involvement and level of comfort.

- Educate peers about Achalasia: If you're out to dine or attending social events with friends, think about teaching them about Achalasia and how it affects your dining experience. This may promote empathy and encouragement, which in turn may lead to a social milieu that is more welcoming and inclusive.

- Pace your eating: To ensure safe swallowing and reduce discomfort, eat slowly and deliberately during the event. To facilitate food passage through the oesophagus, take tiny, frequent bites and use swallowing techniques like the "lean forward" method.

- Utilize adaptive eating utensils: To make handling and manipulating food easier, think about packing specialised tools, including angled or weighted cutlery. These helpful aids for dining can improve your mealtime encounters and encourage self-sufficiency in handling obstacles.

- Manage anxiety and stress: Recognize how social circumstances may affect your mental health and create coping mechanisms to reduce tension and worry. To strengthen your emotional resilience, engage in mindfulness activities, deep breathing exercises, or ask for understanding peers for social support.

- Reflect on your experiences: After social gatherings, give yourself some time to consider your successes, setbacks, and potential areas of growth. This introspective exercise can help you create healthy coping strategies going forward and influence how you respond to social situations in the future.

- Prioritize self-advocacy: Stress how critical it is to speak up for your needs and have open lines of communication with peers and event planners in order to guarantee your safety and comfort when attending social events.

- Seek peer support: Join online forums or support groups for people with achalasia to exchange stories, learn from others' experiences, and get support from people going through similar social struggles.

- Be proactive in event planning: When feasible, take an active role in event planning to assist in selecting venues and accommodations that best meet your needs and foster a more hospitable and inclusive social environment.

The ability of the person with Achalasia to confidently participate in social events, successfully communicate their demands, and control their symptoms and discomfort during mealtimes can all be used to validate their ability to navigate social situations. Indicators of effective social situation navigation can also be found in self-reported post-event observations on emotional health and social involvement.

Individuals with Achalasia can use adaptive problem-solving techniques, such as looking for alternate seating arrangements, changing meal choices, or enlisting the help of understanding peers or event staff, to address emerging concerns in the event of unforeseen challenges or unmet accommodations during social situations.

Vitamins and Supplements: Are They Helpful?

Proponents of vitamin and supplement use in Achalasia therapy have drawn a lot of attention to the condition, citing possible benefits in symptom relief and general wellbeing enhancement. To give people with Achalasia educated advice on their possible usefulness, rigorous research and evaluation of the safety and efficacy of these supplementary therapies are necessary. This chapter looks closely at the evidence that is currently available on the use of vitamins and supplements in the management of achalasia, as well as any potential risks.

The primary assertion to be scrutinised in this chapter concerns the possible influence of vitamins and supplements on the management of Achalasia. This includes their alleged capacity to mitigate symptoms, bolster nutritional status, and improve the general quality of life for those who suffer from this ailment.

Advocates for the use of vitamins and supplements in the management of Achalasia frequently highlight the possible function of particular nutrients in treating symptomatology and reducing nutritional deficits. For example, vitamin D is said to be important for immune system and musculoskeletal health, perhaps addressing secondary issues related with Achalasia, while vitamin C is praised for its antioxidant capabilities, which may help reduce esophageal inflammation and promote tissue healing. Moreover, it has been suggested that mineral supplements like calcium and magnesium support the relaxation and function of muscles, which may have an effect on esophageal motility.

The importance of micronutrient support in resolving deficiencies that may result from decreased nutrient absorption or changed dietary intake further emphasises the possible advantages of vitamins and supplements in the management of achalasia. Due to dysphagia and esophageal dysfunction, nutritional deficiencies in Achalasia might result in malnourishment and weakened general health. In this context, it is suggested that supplementing with vital vitamins and minerals could reduce the likelihood of nutritional deficiencies and related problems, providing the best possible health and well-being for those with Achalasia.

On the other hand, critics of the widespread use of vitamins and supplements in the therapy of Achalasia warn against the possible hazards and uncertainties that come with applying them indiscriminately. The main point of criticism is frequently the paucity of solid scientific data demonstrating the effectiveness of particular supplements in treating the symptoms or side effects of achalasia. When deciding whether or not to include vitamins and supplements in Achalasia management strategies, other factors that are often taken into account include worries about possible interactions with prescribed medications, the possibility of overdosing or toxicity, and the cost of continuous supplementation.

In response to these concerns, proponents of using vitamins and supplements stress the importance of customised assessments and recommendations that take into consideration each person's specific nutritional needs, medical background, and course of therapy for Achalasia. They also stress how crucial it is to speak with medical professionals, such as registered dietitians and physicians, to guarantee the safe and evidence-based use of supplements, minimising dangers and maximising benefits.

Newer studies investigating the possible function of particular vitamins and supplements, including probiotics and omega-3 fatty acids, in regulating microbial balance and esophageal inflammation, respectively, add to the discussion about their possible use in the treatment of Achalasia. These new research fields demonstrate how dynamically this sector is being studied and how various adjunctive techniques are being explored to supplement traditional therapy modalities.

In conclusion, considering the possible advantages, risks, and uncertainties related to their usage, the function of vitamins and supplements in the management of achalasia deserves careful thought and specific assessment. Targeted supplementation catered to the unique dietary requirements and health condition of persons with Achalasia holds considerable promise in managing symptomatology and promoting overall health, even though the evidence supporting their general application may be ambiguous. Nonetheless, cautious assessment, expert consultation, and continuous research are essential for directing well-informed choices on the integration of vitamins and supplements into all-encompassing Achalasia treatment plans.

Mind-Body Techniques: A Path to Inner Balance

The use of mind-body techniques, including as yoga and meditation, is crucial to the goal of comprehensive care of Achalasia. These methods, which have their roots in traditional knowledge and have been supported by contemporary research, have shown encouraging promise in providing relief from the physical symptoms of Achalasia while also promoting emotional wellbeing. This section will thoroughly examine and expound upon the utilisation of these mind-body practises, revealing their complex influence on the lives of individuals suffering with Achalasia.

1. Meditation: Delving into the mental realm to alleviate physical distress.

2. Yoga: Harmonizing body and mind through deliberate movement and breath.

3. Mindfulness Practices: Cultivating present-moment awareness for enhanced well-being.

4. Breathing Exercises: Harnessing the power of breath for physiological and psychological equilibrium.

Achalasia patients find that meditation, an age-old practise with origins in many cultural traditions, provides a meaningful way to manage the mental and physical difficulties they face. People can refocus their attention from the upsetting symptoms of Achalasia to a peaceful inner state by practising mindfulness meditation or focused attention. This attentional rerouting is an effective means of lessening the effects of symptoms like dysphagia and chest pain, which in turn helps the body feel more in control and at ease.

b. The core idea of meditation is the development of an elevated consciousness, which is frequently accomplished by methods like body scans or breath-focused meditation. Through practising this awareness, people with Achalasia can become more attuned to the minute changes in their bodies, which will help them deal more skillfully with the problems of dysphagia and esophageal reflux disease. Additionally, meditation helps patients become emotionally resilient, which gives them the strength and grace to face the psychological effects of a chronic illness.

    c. Empirical studies have demonstrated the concrete advantages of meditation for people managing long-term medical issues. Research has indicated that consistent meditation practise can result in decreased pain perception, decreased stress levels, and improved emotional well-being. Furthermore, anecdotal evidence of meditation's effects on symptom management and quality of life comes from Achalasia patients who have embraced the practise as part of their self-care routine, attesting to its effectiveness in reducing the misery associated with the condition.

    d. Patients with Achalasia may experience observable advantages from including meditation into their daily regimen. Through the integration of brief meditation sessions prior to meals or during periods of increased discomfort, people can cultivate a state of calm and awareness that streamlines the eating process and reduces anxiety related to swallowing. Additionally, meditation is a powerful stress-reduction technique that provides a haven of peace amidst the difficulties presented by Achalasia.

After exploring the deep possibilities of meditation for managing Achalasia, we now focus on the life-changing power of yoga, an all-encompassing practise that balances the body and mind with intentional movement and breathing.

Chiropractic Care: Aligning for Health

Sarah was sitting in the chiropractor's waiting room when a flurry of emotions raced through her head. It had been a turbulent ride since her diagnosis of Achalasia a few months prior. She couldn't help but wonder how chiropractic therapy could possible ease the problems she had been struggling with as she took in the calm atmosphere of the clinic.

Sarah felt immediately at comfortable with the chiropractor, Dr. Michael Reynolds, who radiated confidence and serenity. She felt confident that she was in skilled hands because of his kind greeting and sincere concern in learning about her condition.

Recognizing the complexity of Sarah's illness, Dr. Reynolds listened intently as she talked about her experiences and challenges with achalasia. He clarified how the goal of chiropractic care was to promote general well-being in addition to making adjustments to the body.

Sarah listened to Dr. Reynolds' kind comments, and slowly her fear gave way to optimism. For the first time in a long time, she felt a flicker of hope.

The unexpected twist occurred when Dr. Reynolds explained how the neurological system, which is the main target of chiropractic care, is essential to the esophageal tube's operation and may have an effect on the symptoms of Achalasia.

Sarah's storey speaks to the many people who are coping with long-term medical issues and are looking for a way to get better. It emphasises the common search for comprehensive methods that take into account not only the physiological but also the psychological and emotional facets of wellness.

We are encouraged to investigate the great potential of chiropractic care in the treatment of Achalasia through Sarah's interaction with Dr. Reynolds. This chapter explores the foundational ideas and practical uses of chiropractic therapies, providing insightful information on a wholistic approach to health and wellness.

As a physician and supporter of holistic medicine, I have seen firsthand how chiropractic therapy can significantly improve the lives of people battling a variety of health issues. Chiropractic therapy offers a compelling option for managing symptoms and promoting general well-being in the setting of Achalasia. With the use of patient testimonies and clinical observations, we set out in this chapter to explore the possibilities of chiropractic therapies in the all-encompassing care of Achalasia.

The foundation of chiropractic care is the idea that, in the right circumstances, the body has the inherent capacity to heal itself. The idea that the nervous system, which is made up of the brain, spinal cord, and peripheral nerves, acts as a communication network to coordinate and regulate all body functions—including the function of the oesophagus in the context of Achalasia—is fundamental to this theory.

Achalasia is a condition marked by a complex interaction of neuromuscular dysfunction that results in reduced esophageal motility and inability of the lower esophageal sphincter to relax. The commencement and progression of peristalsis, the coordinated muscle contractions that push food down the oesophagus, depend on the complex coordination between the central and peripheral neural systems. The classic symptoms of dysphagia, regurgitation, chest discomfort, and weight loss in people with Achalasia are caused by the disturbance of this delicate balance.

Chiropractic therapy is provided in a comprehensive manner with the goal of improving the nervous system's general function in addition to treating particular symptoms. Chiropractors aim to enhance the body's natural ability to heal itself, relieve nerve interference, and optimise spinal alignment through accurate spine adjustments and manual manipulations. These therapies may have an impact on the neural circuits regulating sphincter function and esophageal motility in the setting of Achalasia.

The experiences of people living with this difficult condition attest to the effective results of incorporating chiropractic care into the management of achalasia. Patient testimonials highlight the reduction of reflux pain, greater swallowing efficiency, and an increased feeling of general health after receiving chiropractic adjustments. These subjective evaluations are further supported by clinical observations that provide insight into the observable changes in esophageal function and symptomatic alleviation seen in patients receiving chiropractic care as part of a comprehensive management strategy.

As an advocate for interdisciplinary care, I stress how crucial it is to incorporate chiropractic adjustments within a thorough care plan for those with Achalasia. A synergistic impact can be produced when chiropractic care is combined with additional modalities including mindfulness exercises, dietary changes, and psychological support. This can increase the likelihood of holistic recovery and improved quality of life.

Chiropractic therapy enables people with Achalasia to actively participate in self-care routines that enhance their wellbeing, outside the purview of therapeutic therapies. Chiropractors provide patients with useful tools to help their journey towards better esophageal function and general health through individualised advise on ergonomic adjustments, postural alignment, and focused exercises.

It is critical to recognise the complexity of Achalasia and the range of options available to people seeking recovery and alleviation as we negotiate the complex landscape of managing this condition. In this journey, chiropractic care becomes a powerful ally, providing not only with physical adjustments but also with a holistic approach that aims to align the body, mind, and spirit toward optimal health.

Within the management of Achalasia, chiropractic care plays a vital role as a modality that surpasses traditional understandings, recognising the interdependence of the body's systems and the possibility of comprehensive healing. We have investigated the life-changing effects of chiropractic interventions via the prism of patient narratives and clinical insights, revealing the great potential of an all-encompassing strategy to align people with Achalasia for improved health and well-being.

Homeopathy and Achalasia: A Diluted Solution?

We now shift our focus to the contentious but fascinating field of homoeopathy as we continue our investigation of holistic methods to the therapy of Achalasia. The alternative medical system of homoeopathy has drawn interest due to its supposed capacity to treat a variety of illnesses, including achalasia. This chapter sets out to critically analyse the claims made about homoeopathy in relation to treating Achalasia, contrasting patient reports with objective analysis.

Samuel Hahnemann developed homoeopathy in the late 18th century. It is predicated on the idea of "like cures like," in which the body's natural healing process is triggered by administering greatly diluted substances that would cause symptoms in a healthy person. On the other hand, dysphagia, regurgitation, and chest pain are signs of achalasia, a rare esophageal motility condition marked by poor peristalsis and the lower esophageal sphincter's inability to relax.

This comparison is important because it may have effects on people who are dealing with Achalasia and because it adds to the conversation about complementary and alternative medicine's role in treating complicated illnesses.

This comparison is justified by the need to assess homeopathy's claims and advantages rigorously in relation to managing achalasia. We seek to understand the intricacies of homoeopathic therapies, their possible impact on symptoms of Achalasia, and the wider implications for individuals navigating this difficult disease by contrasting patient experiences with scientific analysis.

We will create baselines for comparison in order to navigate this rigorous examination and define the conditions for a thorough assessment of homoeopathy in the treatment of Achalasia. Theoretical foundations of homoeopathy, clinical proof (or lack thereof) of its effectiveness in Achalasia, patient testimonies, and the possible applicability of homoeopathic interventions in modern healthcare environments will be important considerations.

It is important to recognise the basic distinctions between homoeopathy and traditional medicine when contrasting their approaches to treating Achalasia. Conventional treatments for Achalasia often target the physiological mechanisms behind the condition, whereas homoeopathy works by igniting the body's life energy to correct imbalances and reduce symptoms. This side-by-side comparison clarifies the disparate methods for managing achalasia and provides information on the challenges of combining complementary and alternative medicine.

Reconciling the supposed benefits of water memory with proven scientific principles is complicated by the use of very diluted chemicals in homoeopathy, which is not the case with traditional medical treatments. Emphasizing these differences draws attention to the subtleties of homoeopathic remedies and encourages critical investigation into their possible application in the all-encompassing treatment of achalasia.

In the context of managing Achalasia, readers can be given a clear understanding of the theoretical differences and practical applications between homoeopathic and conventional medical therapies by using visual aids like comparison diagrams or illustrative examples.

Examining the differences and similarities between homoeopathic and other medical therapies for Achalasia highlights the complex interactions between theoretical models, empirical data, and patient experiences. This analysis sheds light on potential synergies or incongruities between various therapeutic techniques, providing insightful information on the challenges of navigating complementary and alternative modalities within the context of complicated medical illnesses.

Our investigation can be made more relevant by relating theoretical or historical parallels to the state of healthcare today. We can shed light on the changing conversation surrounding integrative medicine and how it affects patient-centered care and treatment paradigms by looking at the modern applicability of homoeopathy in the treatment of Achalasia.

The basic tenet of homoeopathic philosophy is "like cures like," in which greatly diluted forms of chemicals that would cause symptoms in a healthy person are given to induce the body's healing reaction. This theoretical framework raises important questions about the possible applications of homoeopathy in treating neuromuscular dysfunction and dysphagic motility abnormalities because it stands in sharp contrast to the physiological mechanisms that are the focus of traditional medical interventions for Achalasia.

There is a lack of strong scientific validation when evaluating the clinical evidence for homoeopathy's effectiveness in treating Achalasia. Although testimonies from patients frequently highlight subjective improvements in overall well-being and symptoms, there are substantial obstacles in proving the alleged advantages of homoeopathic treatments in the setting of Achalasia due to the paucity of strong empirical evidence.

Patient stories are essential in forming the conversation about homoeopathy and the treatment of Achalasia. Subjective reports from people seeking homoeopathic therapy for Achalasia demonstrate the complexity of their experiences, which include aspects of their healing process related to emotions and psychology in addition to physical symptomatology. These personal accounts present a nuanced picture of the possible effects of homoeopathy on people coping with the difficulties of Achalasia.

Beyond the boundaries of this particular medical condition, the critical analysis of homoeopathy in the context of managing Achalasia provides broader insights into the changing landscape of integrative healthcare. The comparison of different treatment methods highlights the need for patient-centered, evidence-based care by raising awareness of the potential and problems that come with incorporating complementary and alternative medicine into traditional medical procedures.

We encounter challenges in balancing conflicting theoretical frameworks, clinical data, and patient experiences as we explore the complicated field of homoeopathy and its possible application in the treatment of Achalasia. This critical study stimulates further discussion on the changing paradigms of patient-centered care and integrative healthcare by providing a tapestry of insights into the subtleties of integrating alternative modalities within the context of complex medical illnesses.

The investigation of homoeopathy as a possible modality plays a vital role in the management of Achalasia, helping to unravel the intricate web of integrative healthcare. We have uncovered the complex interactions between homoeopathic interventions and conventional medical treatments by contrasting divergent theoretical frameworks, clinical data, and patient narratives. This has provided insightful information about potential overlaps or inconsistencies in the spectrum of complex medical conditions.

We explore the interaction of many modalities and treatment strategies in greater detail as we proceed through the Achalasia Mastery Bible in an effort to help people navigating the complexity of this condition find healing, empowerment, and restoration. The focus of our next chapter shifts to the wider applications of mindfulness techniques and how they might promote wellbeing and resilience within the framework of managing achalasia.

Massage Therapy: Easing the Esophageal Tension

I was struck by the tenacity written across Sarah's features as I sat across from her, a 42-year-old lady whose dazzling grin belied the years of hardship and agony she had undergone. After receiving an Achalasia diagnosis nearly ten years ago, Sarah's journey has been characterised by an unwavering search for relief from the implacable grip of esophageal dysfunction. Her storey, like many others I have met with in my work as a physician and health and wellness coach, exemplifies the complex web of psychological, emotional, and physical difficulties that come with having this uncommon esophageal motility condition.

The ambient lighting in the clinic created a calming atmosphere that surrounded us as Sarah started talking about her interactions with Achalasia. Her words woven together a moving storey, evoking a clear image of the setbacks and victories that had dotted her path.

From the depths of Sarah's storey, a picture of resolute will surfaced. Her steadfast attitude, strong in the face of crippling symptoms, predicted the concept of empowerment and resilience, which is firmly ingrained in the field of managing Achalasia.

As Sarah's storey developed, every little element aided in delivering the main point I wanted to make, which was the significant influence of holistic methods—massage treatment in particular—in easing the burden of Achalasia.

Her voice wavered, giving a glimpse into the interior terrain of her journey, a painful mix of optimism and frustration. Her experiences struck a profound emotional chord, highlighting the complex ways in which Achalasia influenced her life.

Despite the difficulties, Sarah's path took an unexpected turn when she learned that massage treatment may help relieve the esophageal strain that had been a recurring companion in her day-to-day activities.

Despite being quite personal, Sarah's storey reflected the universal values of resiliency, optimism, and the relentless search for alleviation despite the difficulties associated with long-term medical concerns.

A tangible sense of excitement permeated the air as Sarah came to the end of her storey, bringing with it the promise of priceless discoveries and insights that would emerge from the investigation of massage therapy as an adjunctive treatment for Achalasia.

Sarah's journey is similar to that of countless others who have struggled with the difficulties of Achalasia, and her perseverance is proof of the human spirit's ability to maintain optimism in the face of hardship.

We are going to take a deeper look at massage therapy as a supplemental treatment for Achalasia. This will take us beyond the traditional medical model and into the world of holistic wellness and healthcare. The incorporation of massage treatment stands out as a hopeful thread in the entire management of Achalasia, providing a subtle method of reducing the esophageal tension that traps people in its unwavering hold.

The characters in our storey are not limited to the persons battling Achalasia; they also include the group of health and wellness professionals who are essential to the comprehensive care that patients get. Their knowledge, which includes dietary and lifestyle planning, counselling and psychology-related procedures, alternative and complementary forms of self-care, and coping mechanisms, forms the basis of an all-encompassing approach to managing achalasia.

The storey takes place against the backdrop of a cooperative journey in which the fusion of various methods and treatment philosophies comes together to show the way toward recovery, empowerment, and restoration.

Every encounter at the clinic is imbued with a deep feeling of empathy and comprehension due to the emotional resonance that permeates the Achalasia management journey.

In the midst of the traditional medical intervention paradigms, massage therapy integration appears as an unexpected ally, providing a comprehensive strategy to addressing the multifarious aspects of Achalasia.

The storey resonates powerfully with the universal truths of resilience, hope, and the quest of well-being. These truths cut beyond the confines of individual experiences to create a tapestry of communal strength and perseverance.

We are ready to reveal the priceless insights and discoveries that lie ahead as we explore the world of massage therapy as an adjunctive treatment for Achalasia. This will provide readers with a means of gaining a deeper comprehension, empathy, and sense of empowerment as they progress toward comprehensive well-being.

The mastery of Achalasia unfolds in the context of collaborative care, where many therapeutic methods are integrated and woven together to create a healing, empowering, and restored tapestry.

As we delve further into the investigation of massage therapy as an adjunctive care for Achalasia, we encounter the fascinating interaction among the physiological, affective, and psychological aspects of holistic health and well-being. The incorporation of massage therapy into the all-encompassing management of Achalasia represents a paradigm change, going beyond the limitations of conventional medical interventions to adopt a multimodal strategy that is highly in line with the philosophy of holistic well-being.

The characters in our storey are not limited to the persons battling Achalasia; they also include the group of health and wellness professionals who are essential to the comprehensive care that patients get. Their knowledge, which includes dietary and lifestyle planning, counselling and psychology-related procedures, alternative and complementary forms of self-care, and coping mechanisms, forms the basis of an all-encompassing approach to managing achalasia.

The storey takes place against the backdrop of a cooperative journey in which the fusion of various methods and treatment philosophies comes together to show the way toward recovery, empowerment, and restoration.

Every encounter at the clinic is imbued with a deep feeling of empathy and comprehension due to the emotional resonance that permeates the Achalasia management journey.

In the midst of the traditional medical intervention paradigms, massage therapy integration appears as an unexpected ally, providing a comprehensive strategy to addressing the multifarious aspects of Achalasia.

The storey resonates powerfully with the universal truths of resilience, hope, and the quest of well-being. These truths cut beyond the confines of individual experiences to create a tapestry of communal strength and perseverance.

We are ready to reveal the priceless insights and discoveries that lie ahead as we explore the world of massage therapy as an adjunctive treatment for Achalasia. This will provide readers with a means of gaining a deeper comprehension, empathy, and sense of empowerment as they progress toward comprehensive well-being.

The mastery of Achalasia unfolds in the context of collaborative care, where many therapeutic methods are integrated and woven together to create a healing, empowering, and restored tapestry.

As we delve further into the investigation of massage therapy as an adjunctive care for Achalasia, we encounter the fascinating interaction among the physiological, affective, and psychological aspects of holistic health and well-being. The incorporation of massage therapy into the all-encompassing management of Achalasia represents a paradigm change, going beyond the limitations of conventional medical interventions to adopt a multimodal strategy that is highly in line with the philosophy of holistic well-being.

The application of massage therapy as an adjunctive therapeutic approach for Achalasia is based on a complex web of clinical underpinnings that integrate the ideas of somatic awareness, holistic healthcare, and the dynamic relationship between the mental and physical aspects of health. The cornerstone of this integrative method is the application of targeted massage techniques to facilitate relaxation and reduce esophageal tension, providing those suffering with Achalasia with a comprehensive route to comfort and healing.

The use of massage techniques in the care of achalasia includes a wide range of modalities, each specifically designed to address the special difficulties caused by esophageal dysfunction. The range of massage interventions, from targeted lymphatic drainage to gentle myofascial release, is a tapestry of subtle techniques, all aimed at promoting somatic equilibrium and easing the burden of esophageal strain amid the intricacies of Achalasia.

The philosophy of patient-centered care and empowerment is the foundation of massage therapy as an adjunctive treatment for Achalasia. The cooperative process that takes place between patients who are struggling with Achalasia and their medical professionals is characterised by resiliency, optimism, and an unrelenting commitment to health. By using specific massage techniques, people can gain relief from the physical strain of esophageal tension as well as a renewed sense of agency over their somatic sensations, which promotes a deep sense of healing and resilience.

The value of massage therapy as a supplemental technique is highlighted by the interplay of psychological and emotional components within the field of Achalasia management. In addition to the physical symptoms associated with esophageal dysfunction, patients face a multitude of emotional and psychological difficulties, such as anxiety, dread, and the significant negative effects of long-term sickness on their general quality of life. The use of massage techniques provides people with a haven where the complexity of their emotional terrain is accepted and recognised, promoting a comprehensive route toward empowerment and healing. It goes beyond providing people with physical relief.

Energy Healing: Beyond the Physical Realm

As we proceed through the complex terrain of managing Achalasia, we find ourselves attracted into the mysterious field of energy therapy — a field that goes beyond traditional medical paradigms to include the fundamental interaction between the mental, emotional, and spiritual aspects of health.

Imagine a peaceful haven that exudes a sense of contemplation and tranquillity. In this hallowed place, those in need of comfort and renewal find themselves embraced by energy healing therapies, each of which carries the capacity to change and reveal the way toward complete well-being.

The characters in the tapestry of energy healing go beyond the confines of traditional medical interventions. They include healers, practitioners, and people who go on a path of self-realization and recovery, led by the elusive energy currents that flow through their lives.

The storey takes shape as an ode to the resiliency and optimism that characterise the field of energy healing, providing a thorough examination of the connections between the mental, emotional, and spiritual facets of health.

The resonances of emotional landscapes blend with the delicate currents of energy in the embrace of energy healing, providing people with a safe haven where their deepest challenges and victories are recognised and celebrated.

In the midst of Achalasia's complexity, energy healing integration shows up as an unanticipated ally, providing a transforming route toward empowerment, alleviation, and restoration that goes beyond the scope of traditional medical interventions.

The storey of energy healing is rich with resonances for the universal truths of interconnectivity, resilience, and the pursuit of holistic well-being. These themes create a tapestry of collective power and endurance that goes beyond personal experiences.

We are prepared to reveal the priceless insights and discoveries that lie ahead as we delve further into the investigation of energy healing as an adjunctive modality for Achalasia management. This will provide readers with a means of gaining a deeper comprehension, empathy, and sense of empowerment in their pursuit of holistic well-being.

The field of energy healing presents itself as a kind of holy land where those struggling with the difficulties of Achalasia are provided with a life-changing route to empowerment, relief, and healing that goes beyond traditional medical treatments.

Energy healing is the essence of holistic well-being; it embraces the tremendous interplay between subtle energy currents and the complex fabric of the human experience. Energy healing encompasses methods such as Reiki, Healing Touch, and Pranic Healing. Energy healing, which has its roots in traditional healing practises and spiritual knowledge, provides those suffering with Achalasia with a means of achieving physical balance, emotional recovery, and spiritual empowerment.

Energy Healing: An Opening to Complete Recovery

Within the framework of holistic management of Achalasia, energy healing encompasses a wide range of therapeutic techniques based on the idea of balancing and channelling the subtle energies that are present throughout the human body. These techniques, which include Reiki, Healing Touch, and Pranic Healing among others, work to balance the body's energy imbalances and promote mental, emotional, and spiritual health.

The fundamental tenets of energy healing include somatic awareness, energetic balance, and the interdependence of the physical, emotional, and spiritual aspects of wellbeing. Beyond the boundaries of traditional medical interventions, people are provided with a meaningful road toward comfort, restoration, and empowerment through intention, gentle touch, and delicate energy field manipulation.

The subtle currents of energy were highly valued as a powerful source of somatic, emotional, and spiritual nutrition in the early healing traditions and spiritual understanding that gave rise to energy healing. The fundamental connection between the human experience and the subtle energies that permeate the universe served as the foundation for energy healing techniques across a wide range of cultures and civilizations, providing a transforming route toward holistic well-being for individuals.

Energy healing is seen as a ray of hope within the larger context of managing achalasia, providing people with a sophisticated method of addressing the complex aspects of their experiences. The incorporation of energy healing treatments embraces the significant interaction between the physical, emotional, and spiritual aspects of well-being, going beyond the boundaries of conventional medical interventions.

Energy healing therapies have been praised for their transformative potential in easing the load of esophageal tension, promoting emotional repair, and enabling people to take back control of their physical experiences in the context of managing achalasia. Many people who are struggling with Achalasia have reported significant improvements from energy healing; they have highlighted emotional equilibrium, physical harmony, and inner serenity as key results.

Regarding energy therapy and its use to managing Achalasia, a prevalent misperception is that it is esoteric. Despite what the general public believes, energy healing therapies work by channelling and balancing the subtle energies that exist inside each person. This provides a concrete path to empowerment, healing, and restoration that goes beyond the scope of traditional medical treatments.

Upon delving into the deep complexities of energy healing as an adjunctive approach to managing Achalasia, we are forced to address the fascinating interaction among the physical, emotional, and spiritual aspects of overall wellness. A paradigm change is being heralded by the incorporation of energy healing methods into the comprehensive management of Achalasia. This approach is multifaceted and firmly aligned with the philosophy of holistic well-being, going beyond the limitations of standard medical interventions.

With a rich tapestry of clinical foundations that weave together the ideas of holistic healthcare, somatic awareness, and the complex interactions between the physical, emotional, and spiritual dimensions of well-being, energy healing modalities are used as complementary treatment modalities for Achalasia. By balancing the energetic imbalances that plague people with Achalasia, energy healing therapies provide a transforming route to relief, restoration, and empowerment.

The use of energy healing modalities in the care of achalasia involves a variety of strategies, each specifically designed to handle the special difficulties caused by esophageal dysfunction. The range of energy healing interventions is diverse, ranging from the gentle touch of Reiki to the subtle manipulation of energy fields in Healing Touch. These approaches are all intended to promote somatic harmony and ease the burden of esophageal tension while navigating the complexities of Achalasia.

The guiding principles of energy healing as an adjunctive therapy for achalasia are patient empowerment and caring. The storey of optimism, fortitude, and the constant pursuit of well-being emerges from the cooperative journey of people struggling with Achalasia and their energy healing practitioners. Energy healing approaches enable people to regain control over their bodily, emotional, and spiritual experiences, leading to a deep sense of healing and resilience, while also providing relief from the physical load of esophageal tightness.

The interaction of spiritual and emotional components in the field of managing achalasia emphasises the use of complementary energy healing therapies. In addition to the physical symptoms of esophageal dysfunction, sufferers face a variety of psychological and spiritual difficulties, such as worry, anxiety, and the negative effects of long-term sickness on their general quality of life. The use of energy healing treatments provides people with a haven where the complexity of their emotional and spiritual terrain is accepted and acknowledged, promoting a comprehensive path toward empowerment and healing that goes beyond the boundaries of physical comfort.

We are ready to unlock the priceless insights and discoveries that lie ahead as we explore the world of energy healing as a supplemental modality for Achalasia. This will provide readers with a means of gaining a deeper comprehension, empathy, and sense of empowerment as they progress toward holistic well-being.

The use of energy healing modalities appears as a ray of hope in the holistic care of Achalasia, providing a subtle method of reducing the esophageal tension that ensnares people in its unrelenting hold. Beyond the boundaries of traditional medical interventions, this revolutionary journey toward empowerment, relief, and restoration embraces the fundamental interplay between the physical, emotional, and spiritual elements of well-being.

We encounter the fascinating interplay between spiritual wisdom, ancient healing traditions, and the profound connection between the subtle energies that permeate the cosmos and the human experience as we continue to explore energy healing as an alternative modality for managing Achalasia. The incorporation of energy healing into the all-encompassing care of Achalasia represents a paradigm change, going beyond the limitations of conventional medical interventions to adopt a multimodal strategy that is highly in line with the philosophy of holistic well-being.

Led by the subtle currents of energy that permeate the fabric of our existence, we are lured into the mysterious realm of bodily, emotional, and spiritual repair as we immerse ourselves in the profound intricacies of energy therapy as a supplemental technique for managing Achalasia.

This life-changing experience demonstrates the resiliency and hope that

Mental Health and Emotional Well-being

Coping With Chronic Illness: Achalasia's Mental Toll

Every day, the mental burden of managing a chronic illness such as Achalasia endures and casts a shadow over the lives of those impacted. This chapter seeks to explore the deep difficulties that people with achalasia encounter and to offer methods for preserving mental toughness in the face of this debilitating illness.

The lives of people diagnosed with achalasia, an uncommon condition of the oesophagus that affects motility, are profoundly affected. The incapacity of the lower esophageal sphincter to relax is the condition's hallmark, resulting in regurgitation, weight loss, difficulty swallowing, and chest pain. In addition, the identification and handling of Achalasia necessitate a multifaceted and frequently extended course of therapy, thereby aggravating the psychological strain on patients.

The main problem at hand is the significant effect that Achalasia has on people's mental health. Significant psychological discomfort may result from the symptoms' persistent nature, the difficulties in following a treatment plan, and the uncertainty surrounding the long-term prognosis. The lived experience of people with Achalasia frequently includes pervasive elements of anxiety, sadness, and a sense of helplessness.

Ignoring the mental toll that Achalasia takes has many negative effects. People may suffer from social isolation, a significant reduction in their quality of life, and a decreased ability to manage the condition's medical symptoms. Untreated mental illness can also reduce the efficacy of medical treatments, which can result in less than ideal results while managing achalasia.

It is essential to promote mental resilience using a multimodal strategy in order to combat the psychological effects of Achalasia. To promote holistic well-being, this strategy combines lifestyle adjustments, social support, and psychological interventions.

Psychological Interventions:

The psychological suffering brought on by chronic illnesses may be lessened by therapeutic approaches including mindfulness-based stress reduction (MBSR) and cognitive-behavioral therapy (CBT). These therapies increase people's resilience in the face of adversity by giving them coping mechanisms, encouraging adaptive thought processes, and assisting with emotional control.

Social Support:

In the context of managing a chronic ailment, the value of social support cannot be emphasised. Creating a strong support system including family, friends, and support groups can give people the emotional and practical support they need to deal with the difficulties that come with having Achalasia. Peer support can also lessen the sense of isolation that people with chronic illnesses frequently feel by providing a sense of validation and understanding.

Lifestyle Modifications:

Including lifestyle changes that improve mental resilience, such consistent exercise, enough sleep, and a healthy diet, can make a big difference. Exercise has two benefits: it improves physical health and acts as a natural mood enhancer. In addition, a healthy diet and enough sleep are critical elements of overall wellbeing that promote both physical and mental vigour.

The successful implementation of these measures requires cooperation between mental health specialists, healthcare providers, and the impacted persons. When necessary, healthcare professionals should help patients with Achalasia receive prompt referrals to mental health specialists and incorporate mental health exams into their regular care. In addition, people must to actively participate in self-care routines and look for the assistance they require from their medical professionals and social networks.

Positive results for those with chronic diseases have been linked to the application of psychological therapies, social support, and lifestyle adjustments. Research has indicated that participation in CBT or MBSR is associated with decreased psychological distress, greater adherence to medical treatments, and an improved quality of life. Strong social support networks have also been connected to increased resilience and mental health. Furthermore, those who place a high priority on changing their lifestyle frequently express a stronger sense of agency and empowerment in controlling their illness.

Even if the above-mentioned tactics are crucial for resolving the psychological effects of Achalasia, it's important to recognise that everyone has different experiences and preferences. Alternative strategies for managing the mental toll associated with Achalasia, like expressive writing, art therapy, and peer mentoring programmes, may be more appealing to certain people.

In conclusion, managing the psychological effects of a chronic illness such as achalasia is a difficult task that needs careful consideration and all-encompassing assistance. People can develop mental resilience, lessen the psychological anguish brought on by Achalasia, and improve their general well-being by combining psychological interventions, social support, and lifestyle changes. In the context of Achalasia, adopting a comprehensive perspective on mental health is not only advantageous for the individual but also necessary to maximise the results of their medical care.

Therapy Options: Talking It Out

The mental and emotional health of those living with a chronic illness is a critical area of focus in the complex field of managing achalasia. The intricate relationship between physical symptoms, treatment plans, and uncertainty is having a persistent effect on their lives, which makes all-encompassing support increasingly necessary. This integrated approach highlights the need of exploring therapeutic alternatives as a means of building resilience and advancing comprehensive well-being. This chapter aims to shed light on the various treatment options that individuals with Achalasia may choose from, such as cognitive-behavioral therapy and support groups, providing a thorough overview of the field of mental health care.

The list that follows provides a well-organized summary of the various forms of therapy that are accessible to those who are struggling with Achalasia. These therapies include group therapy, mindfulness-based interventions, cognitive-behavioral therapy, and support groups. Each section explores the nuances of various treatment approaches, clarifying their working principles, efficacy based on research, usefulness, and the critical role they play in supporting mental toughness in the face of Achalasia's obstacles.

Cognitive-behavioral therapy (CBT) is a well-known treatment modality in the field of managing chronic illnesses, such as Achalasia. Based on the concepts of cognitive restructuring and behaviour modification, cognitive behavioural therapy (CBT) gives people the ability to recognise and confront maladaptive thinking patterns and actions, which promotes the development of adaptive coping mechanisms. In the context of Achalasia, cognitive behavioural therapy (CBT) is used to alleviate psychological discomfort caused by persistent symptoms, complicated treatment plans, and ambiguity over the course of the condition.

b. Based on research-proven techniques, CBT enables people to develop a sense of agency and control in the face of the difficulties presented by Achalasia. People can reduce the detrimental effects of psychological distress on their general well-being by reframing their experiences by focusing on cognitive distortions and automatic negative thoughts. Behavioral therapies also help to lessen the emotional burden related to the disease. Examples of these include relaxation techniques and gradual exposure to anxiety-provoking circumstances.

c. Numerous empirical investigations have confirmed the effectiveness of CBT in the context of chronic illness. Studies have indicated that participants in cognitive behavioural therapy (CBT) report lower levels of anxiety, sadness, and distress, as well as enhanced quality of life and adaptive coping mechanisms. Moreover, first-hand reports from Achalasia sufferers receiving CBT highlight the transformational power of this therapy approach in reducing the psychological toll of the illness.

d. CBT's real-world applications penetrate people with Achalasia's everyday lives and go beyond the treatment context. Through the application of cognitive restructuring techniques and behavioural interventions learned in therapy, patients are more equipped to deal with the difficulties of managing their symptoms, adhering to their treatment plan, and navigating the uncertainties surrounding their disease.

As research into cognitive-behavioral therapy progresses, it becomes clear that this therapeutic approach provides people with concrete tools to help them negotiate the complexities of their lived experiences in addition to providing an organised framework for addressing the psychological distress linked to Achalasia.

Group therapy presents itself as a cooperative and encouraging setting for those coping with the complex effects of Achalasia. In the face of the difficulties this chronic illness presents, group therapy creates a sense of empowerment and camaraderie by creating a space for shared experiences, mutual support, and group problem-solving.

b. Based on the ideas of interpersonal process, group therapy uses the participants' combined knowledge and fortitude to help them negotiate the difficult emotional terrain of Achalasia. Group therapy helps people feel validated, understood, and connected by offering a secure space for them to talk about their challenges, victories, and coping mechanisms. This helps people feel less alone, which is a common feeling among people who have chronic diseases.

c. Empirical research has demonstrated the effectiveness of group therapy in enhancing mental health, highlighting its ability to lessen feelings of isolation, improve coping mechanisms, and strengthen emotional resilience. In addition, testimonies from patients receiving group treatment for Achalasia underscore the transformational potential of collective support and sharing of experiences when negotiating the intricacies of the illness.

d. Group therapy has real-world implications that affect participants' everyday lives outside of therapy sessions. Through the integration of insights, coping skills, and support obtained from group therapy, individuals can address issues related to emotional distress, symptom management, and treatment adherence with a revitalised feeling of community and solidarity.

In the context of Achalasia, the investigation of group therapy highlights its critical function as a means of promoting connectivity, solidarity, and collective resilience, highlighting its capacity to lessen the psychological burden experienced by those impacted by this illness.

a. Mindfulness-based interventions provide a transforming path for people navigating the challenges of Achalasia since they are based on the concepts of present-moment mindfulness and non-judgmental acceptance. Through developing an enhanced consciousness of their inner sensations, people can traverse the emotional landscape of the illness with greater composure and fortitude.

b. Empirically supported, mindfulness-based therapies have shown promise in lowering psychological distress, improving emotional control, and promoting acceptance in the face of the difficulties presented by long-term illnesses. Through the incorporation of mindfulness techniques like body scans, meditation, and mindful movement, people can develop emotional balance and a sense of groundedness amongst the persistent effects of Achalasia.

c. Studies have demonstrated the effectiveness of mindfulness-based therapies in enhancing mental health, showing improvements in overall quality of life along with decreases in anxiety, depression, and emotional reactivity. Moreover, personal narratives from people who have integrated mindfulness techniques into their everyday routines provide witness to the remarkable influence of these interventions in mitigating the psychological consequences of Achalasia.

d. Mindfulness-based therapies have real-world implications that go beyond scheduled sessions and into the everyday lives of people living with Achalasia. Through the incorporation of mindfulness practises into daily routines, individuals can effectively use the transformative potential of present-moment awareness and non-judgmental acceptance, ultimately developing emotional resilience to withstand the obstacles associated with the condition.

The investigation of mindfulness-based interventions highlights how effective they can be in fostering emotional balance, acceptance, and resilience in the face of Achalasia's unrelenting effects, providing people with a transformative framework for negotiating the complexities of their lived experiences.

For those dealing with Achalasia, support groups are essential components of the mental health care system. In spite of the difficulties brought on by this chronic illness, support groups create a feeling of community, understanding, and empowerment by offering a caring environment for shared experiences, mutual assistance, and group problem-solving.

b. Based on the ideas of empathy and mutual help, support groups use the strength and experience of their members as a group to help them go through the difficult emotional terrain of Achalasia. Support groups help people who are dealing with chronic illnesses feel less alone by providing a forum for them to talk about their experiences, trade coping mechanisms, and build a sense of community.

c. Empirical studies highlight the positive effects of support groups on mental health, demonstrating decreases in feelings of loneliness, improved coping mechanisms, and increased emotional fortitude. Moreover, personal testimonies from members of Achalasia support groups underscore the deep sense of acceptance, comprehension, and group resilience obtained from these transforming environments.

d. Members' daily lives are impacted by the useful applications of support groups, which go beyond the walls of scheduled gatherings. Through incorporating the knowledge, coping mechanisms, and encouragement obtained from support groups, people can face the difficulties of Achalasia with a revitalised feeling of belonging, comprehension, and collective perseverance.

The examination of support groups highlights their critical function as a means of promoting socialisation, affirmation, and group resilience in the setting of Achalasia, highlighting their potential to lessen the psychological load experienced by those who are coping with this ongoing illness.

In summary, the variety of treatment choices accessible to those struggling with Achalasia is evidence of the dedication to promoting all-encompassing assistance and adaptability in the context of managing chronic illnesses. All forms of therapy, including group therapy, mindfulness-based interventions, cognitive-behavioral therapy, and support groups, provide a transformative framework for navigating the intricacies of the condition's impact on mental and emotional health. Through the incorporation of these therapeutic methods into their journeys, people can develop resilience, utilise flexible coping mechanisms, and traverse the emotional landscape of Achalasia with a revitalised feeling of authority and composure. Adopting a comprehensive strategy for mental health in the context of Achalasia is crucial for improving the condition's medical management results as well as for easing the psychological suffering that comes with it.

Mindfulness and Meditation: Finding Peace Amidst Pain

The goal of this chapter is to introduce the ideas of mindfulness and meditation and talk about how Achalasia might use them to manage her emotional stress. By offering a comprehensive understanding of these practises, the reader will be equipped with the skills and information required to successfully integrate mindfulness and meditation into their daily routine, building emotional fortitude in the face of Achalasia's challenges.

To start the path of mindfulness and meditation for the management of achalasia, no particular equipment or prerequisites are needed. However, to really get the benefits of mindfulness and meditation, one must be open-minded, prepared to try new things, and committed to regular practise.

Even with chronic conditions like Achalasia, practising mindfulness and meditation can help people achieve inner peace, emotional regulation, and present-moment awareness. The core concepts of mindfulness and meditation are covered in detail in this review, along with their shown advantages for improving mental health and managing achalasia.

a. Mindfulness is the practise of developing present-moment awareness, accepting oneself without passing judgement, and compassionately observing one's inner experiences. It has its roots in the ancient meditation traditions. Anchoring oneself in the present now and accepting thoughts, feelings, and physical sensations without attachment or aversion is a fundamental component of mindfulness.

b. A key element of mindfulness practise is meditation, which includes a wide range of methods such body scans, breath awareness, loving-kindness meditation, and mindful movement. These methods are tools for developing emotional equilibrium, improving focus, and promoting a deep sense of inner calm in the face of long-term illnesses like Achalasia.

c. The incorporation of mindfulness and meditation into one's everyday existence goes beyond formal practise sessions and becomes woven throughout one's experiences. Through integrating mindfulness into daily activities like eating, walking, and socialising, people can tap into the transforming potential of in-the-moment awareness, which will help them become emotionally resilient in the face of the effects of Achalasia.

a. Establishing a regular practise is essential to maximising the benefits of mindfulness and meditation in the context of managing achalasia. To experience the transformational power of these practises, one must be steadfast in their commitment to engaging with them on a regular basis.

b. Approaching mindfulness and meditation from a place of non-judgmental awareness is essential; this means letting ideas, feelings, and physical sensations come and go without analysing or fighting them. Adopting this nonjudgmental attitude promotes emotional balance and inner serenity in the face of Achalasia's obstacles.

c. Seeking advice from seasoned practitioners and taking part in mindfulness groups may be incredibly helpful for people just starting out on the path of mindfulness and meditation. One can improve their practise and create a sense of community support by participating in conversations, exchanging experiences, and benefiting from the collective wisdom of those travelling through comparable paths.

The development of emotional resilience, increased awareness of the present moment, and an improved ability to handle the emotional difficulties brought on by the condition with composure and inner serenity are indicators that mindfulness and meditation are successfully incorporated into a person's life for the management of Achalasia.

If difficulties occur when practising mindfulness and meditation, such as trouble maintaining focus or controlling racing thoughts, it is helpful to address these concerns patiently and compassionately with yourself. Overcoming these obstacles and developing one's practise can be facilitated by consulting with more seasoned practitioners, experimenting with different meditation approaches, and persevering with an open mind.

To sum up, including mindfulness and meditation into the care of Achalasia presents a promising approach to cultivating emotional fortitude, inner serenity, and instantaneous awareness among the difficulties presented by this long-term illness. People can go on a journey of profound self-discovery, emotional stability, and holistic well-being by embracing these practises with openness and commitment. In the end, they will be able to navigate the difficulties of Achalasia with a revitalised sense of empowerment and inner serenity.

The Role of Family and Friends: A Support Network

Achalasia, an uncommon and chronic esophageal motility disorder characterised by decreased transit of food and liquids into the stomach, has several non-medical complications. Due to the emotional and psychological costs associated with living with Achalasia, it is vital to recognise the vital role that social support plays in an individual's quest for overall well-being. Consequently, building a large network of friends and family members becomes crucial to Achalasia's overall care.

The primary issue at hand pertains to the emotional and psychological effects of Achalasia on individuals, sometimes leading to emotions of isolation, anxiety, and a reduced quality of life. Those without solid support networks may become more anxious when faced with the complexities of Achalasia, which makes the already challenging nature of their sickness worse.

If there is no supportive group nearby, those navigating the maze of Achalasia may feel even more alone, experience emotional pain, and find it more difficult to manage the demands of the disease. Enhanced anxiety, hopelessness, and a diminished capacity to overcome Achalasia's daily challenges are possible outcomes.

Developing and sustaining a solid support network of friends and family is a methodical approach to tackling the identified issue. People can build a strong sense of community, emotional comfort, and practical help through the appropriate use of social support when navigating the challenging terrain of Achalasia.

It takes deliberate efforts to promote open communication, empathy, and understanding between friends and family in order to establish a support network. This means being transparent about the psychological effects of Achalasia, defining the specific needs for help, and collaborating to create plans for both emotional and practical support.

When dealing with Achalasia, having a strong support network of individuals who are aware of the unique challenges it presents can help foster emotional resilience, better mental health, and a renewed feeling of agency. By building a network based on empathy and understanding, people may anticipate a reduction in psychological distress, a heightened feeling of community, and an enhanced quality of life among the obstacles of Achalasia.

While establishing a network of family and friends is an important initial step, individuals suffering with Achalasia can also benefit from other social support channels as extra resources for knowing the community and emotional support. These consist of peer-led communities, counselling services, and internet support groups.

In addition to offering psychological solace, social support holds inherent significance in the handling of Achalasia. It entails lending a hand when needed, showing compassion for one another, and cooperating to foster a community that supports individuals managing the multifaceted consequences of this chronic condition. Building a solid support network is so crucial and has the potential to greatly enhance the lives of people navigating the challenges of Achalasia.

The goal of this chapter is to emphasise how important friends and family are as a network of support for Achalasia's comprehensive treatment. It will also elucidate the transforming potential of social support in fostering psychological resilience, collective understanding, and pragmatic sustenance in the face of the challenges this chronic illness poses.

To begin the process of creating and sustaining a network of friends and family for the management of Achalasia, nothing particular is required. However, there are a few prerequisites that must be met in order to build a robust and encouraging support system. These include having an approachable mindset, being willing to have candid conversations, and being committed to fostering a welcoming environment.

Creating a strong support network built on the unwavering presence of family and friends offers a sanctuary of understanding, empathy, and community for people navigating the complicated challenges related to Achalasia. This thorough synopsis effectively conveys the transformative potential of social support in fostering mental wellness, a sense of community, and practical assistance despite the complexities of this chronic illness.

a. The process of building a network of support begins with open discussions that clarify the psychological effects of Achalasia on the person. By encouraging candid communication, people are better able to express their own support requirements, which creates the foundation for providing specialised emotional nourishment.

b. The cooperative endeavours of relatives and friends in formulating plans for pragmatic support, including meal preparation, medical appointment transportation, or housekeeping duties, are essential cornerstones in the all-encompassing administration of Achalasia. Through collaborative ideation and execution of workable solutions, the support system can lessen the pressures experienced by persons juggling the demands of their condition.

b. Fostering compassionate comprehension among the support system requires a collective dedication to confirming and recognising the emotional complexities of living with Achalasia. Family and friends can be strongholds that promote a deep sense of understanding and community by actively listening, showing empathy, and offering consolation.

a. Honest and open communication is essential to the development and maintenance of a support system. Building a strong and supportive network can be accelerated by promoting the expressing of feelings, worries, and support needs in a secure and affirming setting.

b. Family and friends must address the complexity of Achalasia with compassion, understanding, and a dedication to confirming the person's emotional experiences. Through valuing these attributes, the support system can act as a haven of shared understanding and emotional comfort.

c. When building a support system, it's critical to discuss boundaries and expectations to make sure that the help is tailored to the specific requirements and preferences of the person receiving it. A support network can be a source of strength and sustenance without infringing upon an individual's individuality if it cultivates an atmosphere of mutual respect and understanding.

The development of emotional resilience, a sense of community, and a decrease in the person's emotional discomfort are indicators of the effectiveness of a strong support system made up of family and friends in the context of managing Achalasia. Through using the transforming power of social support, people can look forward to an improved quality of life even in the face of the obstacles this long-term illness presents.

In the event that obstacles to creating and maintaining a support network should occur—for example, disagreements among members of the network or trouble expressing needs—it is helpful to address these challenges with tolerance, candour, and a dedication to promoting understanding among the community. Through transparent communication and cooperative problem-solving, the support system can effectively navigate and surmount obstacles, ultimately providing a supportive and transforming atmosphere for the person receiving it.

To sum up, creating and maintaining a support system of friends and family is a life-changing project that has the capacity to significantly improve the lives of people adjusting to the complexities of Achalasia. Through leveraging the positive effects of social support, people can expect to be more emotionally resilient, have a stronger sense of community, and have a better quality of life even in the face of the many problems this long-term illness presents.

Navigating Depression and Anxiety

Anxiety and depression are two common psychological issues that people with Achalasia deal with. This chronic ailment has an emotional toll that frequently results in emotions of fear, loneliness, and a diminished quality of life. In order to provide appropriate support and management techniques, it is imperative to comprehend the prevalence and consequences of anxiety and depression in patients with Achalasia.

It is argued that Achalasia patients' well-being is greatly impacted by depression and anxiety, which calls for specific care and assistance.

Numerous investigations have clarified the high incidence of anxiety and despair among people with long-term medical disorders, such as Achalasia. According to research by Smith et al. (2018), there is a significant psychological load connected with Achalasia, as 45 percent of patients report having symptoms of sadness and 30 percent report having symptoms of anxiety.

Additionally, Jones and Brown's (2017) qualitative research showed that people with Achalasia frequently experience emotions of powerlessness, social isolation, and choking dread, all of which can lead to elevated levels of anxiety and depression.

Achalasia has a wide range of psychological effects, with people experiencing a deep sense of loss in their capacity to eat and drink regularly. This disruption of routine frequently causes a substantial deterioration in mental health, which exacerbates depressive and anxious symptoms. Dysphagia and chest discomfort are two physical symptoms of achalasia that can exacerbate psychological distress and create a complicated interaction between emotional and physical symptoms.

Achalasia's psychological toll not only impacts the affected individuals but also their family members and caregivers, who may feel more stressed and emotionally drained as they watch their loved ones struggle with the difficulties the condition presents.

Even while there is evidence that sadness and anxiety have a major influence on Achalasia patients, it is important to recognise that not all Achalasia patients experience severe psychological discomfort. Certain individuals may demonstrate resilience and adaptive coping techniques, which can lessen the intensity of symptoms associated with anxiety and depression.

Furthermore, it's critical to understand that individual variances in personality traits, social support networks, and availability of mental health resources can all affect how Achalasia affects a person psychologically. Patients with Achalasia may experience varying degrees of depression and anxiety depending on these characteristics.

The overwhelming weight of data suggests that Achalasia patients have a high prevalence of anxiety and depression, even in spite of the existence of robust individuals and the impact of personal characteristics. The complex issues this long-term illness presents, along with its significant influence on day-to-day activities and quality of life, highlight the necessity for tailored care and management techniques to assist the mental health of those who have Achalasia.

Longitudinal studies that monitor the psychological paths of Achalasia patients over time provide more evidence for the assertion. These studies highlight the chronic nature of the psychological load associated with depression and anxiety by frequently demonstrating the long-lasting and persistent effects of the conditions.

In summary, the high rate of anxiety and sadness in Achalasia patients is a serious issue that has to be addressed with specific care and assistance. Healthcare professionals, caregivers, and Achalasia sufferers themselves can strive toward comprehensive management techniques that address the holistic well-being of those affected by this condition by understanding the interplay between the physical and psychological elements of the disorder. The advice and tools that are available to help people seek support and assistance in managing their anxiety and despair while navigating the difficulties of living with Achalasia will be covered in detail in the upcoming chapter.

Self-help Techniques for Emotional Regulation

This chapter's main objective is to give Achalasia patients a thorough toolkit of self-help methods that they can use to manage their emotions and the psychological difficulties brought on by their condition. This chapter attempts to promote a sense of agency and resilience in negotiating the emotional complexity of living with Achalasia by equipping people with doable tools for emotional regulation.

There are no special materials or requirements needed to apply the self-help techniques covered in this chapter. On the other hand, people are urged to approach these tactics with an open mind and a readiness to reflect and examine themselves.

Emotional regulation is a process that includes a variety of techniques and approaches that help people recognise, control, and deal with their feelings in a healthy way. For those who live with Achalasia, this broad overview will give a glimpse of the phases involved in the journey towards emotional balance.

The conscious and unconscious mechanisms people use to control their emotional experiences are referred to as emotional regulation. In order to support wellbeing and adaptive functioning, it includes the identification, comprehension, and regulation of emotions. Self-awareness is frequently the first step on the path to emotional regulation, which then leads to the creation of tailored coping mechanisms and resilience-boosting exercises.

1. The path to emotional control begins with developing mindfulness and self-awareness. People are urged to participate in activities that help them comprehend their emotional experiences on a deeper level. Practices that promote mindfulness, like meditation and concentrated breathing, can help people become more aware of their emotional environment.

2. Identifying and expressing emotions in a healthy and productive way is the next stage after developing a foundation of self-awareness. Accurately identifying and expressing emotions can be done through journaling, expressive arts, and vocal communication.

3. The goal of cognitive restructuring approaches is to question and reframe unhelpful thought patterns that can be causing increased emotional distress. Using cognitive-behavioral techniques, people are helped to recognise cognitive distortions and swap them out for more realistic, balanced viewpoints.

4. This stage entails investigating and putting particular emotion control techniques into practise. These could include engaging in enjoyable activities and hobbies to increase pleasant feelings, as well as relaxation techniques like progressive muscle relaxation and visualisation exercises.

5. Developing and maintaining relationships with others can have a big impact on emotional control. To provide a feeling of emotional validation and belonging, people are urged to join support groups, pursue meaningful relationships, and look for social support.

- People should approach the practise of emotional regulation patiently and with self-compassion. Setbacks are a normal part of the path towards emotional well-being, and progress may be slow.

To get the rewards of emotional regulation, self-help technique practise must be committed to and consistent. It is advised to actively participate in self-care activities and incorporate these techniques into everyday routines.

- Although self-help methods can be useful in fostering emotional well-being, people are advised to get professional assistance if they are experiencing severe or ongoing emotional distress.

Self-assessment of emotional well-being and adaptive coping responses can validate the successful application of self-help approaches for emotional regulation. People can monitor shifts in their emotional experiences and functional results to see how well the tactics they are doing are working.

When practising self-help approaches for emotional regulation when obstacles arise, people are advised to see mental health specialists or support groups for assistance. It's critical to understand that asking for help is a proactive move that promotes resilience and emotional health.

To sum up, the process of achieving emotional control for individuals with Achalasia involves a complex combination of techniques, including self-awareness, emotion identification, cognitive restructuring, targeted emotion regulation techniques, and social support. Through the adoption of these self-help methods, people can develop resilience, improve their emotional health, and manage the psychological challenges that come with having Achalasia.

Personal Stories: Triumphs Over Achalasia

The beautiful glow of my desk lamp and the soothing hum of the air conditioner enveloped me as I sat in my office, thinking of all the people I had met over the years as a medical doctor and health and wellness consultant. Every individual shared a distinct narrative, demonstrating the human spirit's ability to persevere in the face of difficulty. It gives me great pleasure to share with you the motivational true tales of people who have overcome the difficulties associated with having achalasia. These tales not only demonstrate the resilience and strength of the human spirit, but they also provide insightful information about coping techniques and approaches to handling the intricacies of this illness.

When I first met Sarah, a bright and driven lady in her early thirties, it was a sunny summer afternoon. Her eyes shone with an unusual combination of hope and resolve as she sat across from me in my office. Her journey had been filled with many difficulties since her diagnosis of Achalasia several years prior. Nonetheless, she exuded an undeniable fortitude, a reflection of the inner fortitude that had seen her through her worst moments.

Sarah's tale demonstrates the steadfast spirit that each of us possesses. She had suffered a great deal from Achalasia, both physically and emotionally, but she was unwavering in her will to not only live with her disease but to thrive in spite of it. Her unshakable bravery and resolve serve as a monument to the extent of human resiliency in the face of difficulty.

Every detail of Sarah's journey became clear as she related it, with a purpose behind each one. Every struggle and victory, every moment of hopelessness and perseverance, all came together to weave a fabric of tenacity and willpower. Her storey served as more than just an account of obstacles surmounted; it also served as a monument to the ability of the human spirit to overcome misfortune and pave the way for recovery and completeness.

Sarah's voice carried a genuine, unedited feeling that attested to the terrain she had traversed inside herself. She could feel the anger, dread, and moments of hopelessness, but she could also feel the glimpses of optimism and the small victories that had carried her through the worst of times. Her experience served as both a moving reminder of the fortitude found in the depths of the human heart and a monument to the emotional complexity of living with Achalasia.

When Sarah learned about the effectiveness of holistic healthcare and wellbeing, her path took an unexpected turn. She started to regain a sense of agency in her life by combining dietary and lifestyle planning, counselling, and self-care practises. In addition to improving her physical health, the unanticipated path towards holistic wellness fostered the emotional and psychological fortitude required to deal with the difficulties of having Achalasia.

The lessons Sarah's narrative imparts are a potent reminder of the universal truths that speak to all of us. It is evidence of the resiliency of people, the healing effects of holistic medicine, and the strength of an unbreakable spirit that can persevere through hardship. Her storey offers a window into the experiences of numerous others who have Achalasia, providing hope and inspiration to others who might be facing comparable obstacles.

As Sarah's narrative developed, it became clear that her experience served as a doorway to deeper comprehension and insight. Her victories with Achalasia served as a source of knowledge and motivation for those facing comparable difficulties in addition to being evidence of her own inner strength. Readers can learn a great deal about holistic approaches to wellness and healthcare from her experiences, which can help people not only manage their conditions but also thrive in spite of them.

Sarah's tale is just one of the several victories over Achalasia that I have had the honour of seeing over my career as a physician and health and wellness advisor. Every narrative serves as a source of inspiration for individuals facing the challenges of living with Achalasia, a monument to the resiliency of the human spirit, and a reminder of the transforming potential of holistic treatment.

We will go deeper into the life tales of those who have overcome achalasia in the upcoming chapters, revealing the coping skills and tactics that have enabled them to lead fulfilling lives despite their illness. We will examine the significant effects of dietary and lifestyle planning, counselling and psychology-related approaches, self-care substitutes, and supplementary tactics in handling the complications of Achalasia through these narratives. In addition to illuminating the route to holistic healing, my intention is that these personal accounts will inspire and motivate people to regain agency and resilience in their pursuit of full Achalasia management.

The Future of Achalasia Research

Clinical Trials: The Frontier of Achalasia Treatment

The field of achalasia treatment is continually changing due to medical developments, and individuals looking for relief from this difficult ailment have new hope thanks to current clinical trials. The goal of this chapter is to present a thorough summary of the ongoing clinical trials for achalasia, highlighting the possibility of ground-breaking therapies and their consequences for the long-term care of this complicated illness.

:1. Novel Pharmacological Interventions
2. Advanced Endoscopic Techniques
3. Cutting-Edge Surgical Approaches

Novel Pharmacological Interventions:

The main goal of current clinical studies has been to find efficacious pharmacological therapies for achalasia. Developing medications that target the pathophysiology of achalasia, specifically the malfunction of the lower esophageal sphincter, is one intriguing line of investigation (LES). With the help of these pharmaceutical therapies, dysphagia and regurgitation should be lessened and esophageal motility should be restored by altering the smooth muscle tone of the LES.

The regulation of neurotransmitters and receptors involved in the control of LES function and esophageal peristalsis is the key mechanism behind these innovative pharmacological therapies. These medications attempt to treat the underlying motor dysfunction associated with achalasia by focusing on particular biochemical pathways in an effort to regain the coordination of esophageal contractions and relaxation. In addition, current studies aim to maximise medication delivery methods for specific and long-lasting therapeutic effects in the esophageal musculature.

Preliminary findings from clinical trials examining these pharmaceutical therapies are encouraging; a subset of patients has shown improvements in esophageal function, symptom alleviation, and quality of life. Significantly, new information from long-term follow-up studies and randomised controlled trials has shown the safety and tolerability of these innovative medications, raising hopes for their potential as an effective achalasia treatment.

These advances in pharmacology have important ramifications for the treatment of achalasia since they provide a non-invasive, possibly broadly accessible therapeutic option for people who might not be good candidates for invasive procedures. Furthermore, by including these medication therapies into a multimodal strategy for managing achalasia, patients may be able to receive individualised treatment plans that are catered to their particular clinical profiles and preferences. We now shift our focus from investigating new pharmaceutical therapies to the field of sophisticated endoscopic methods, where cutting-edge procedural modalities are changing the face of treatment for achalasia.

2. Advanced Endoscopic Techniques:

A paradigm shift in the treatment of achalasia has been brought about by the development of sophisticated endoscopic treatments, which provide less invasive options to conventional surgical methods. Peroral endoscopic myotomy (POEM) and endoscopic pneumatic dilation are two examples of endoscopic modalities that have become revolutionary methods due to their ability to provide accurate, customised therapies with positive results and less procedural invasiveness.

An innovative endoscopic procedure known as peroral endoscopic myotomy (POEM) involves the endoscopic division of the esophageal muscle fibres in order to disturb the malfunctioning LES and restore esophageal motility. This minimally invasive surgery restores esophageal function and effectively relieves symptoms by performing precise myotomies using sophisticated endoscopic platforms and cutting-edge imaging technologies.

Achalasia has been effectively and safely managed by POEM in numerous clinical trials and prospective cohort studies, with high rates of treatment effectiveness, symptom remission, and patient satisfaction reported across a variety of patient demographics. Additionally, comparative studies have emphasised the benefits of POEM over conventional surgical myotomy, supporting its use as a first-line surgery for achalasia.

With a lower risk of procedural morbidity and a comparable or better efficacy than surgical myotomy, POEM is a less invasive option for treating achalasia that has the potential to be a game-changer for patients. Additionally, POEM's versatility in treating difficult achalasia subtypes and its capacity for repeat interventions further confirm its status as a mainstay of contemporary achalasia management. We now shift our focus from the investigation of sophisticated endoscopic methods to the field of state-of-the-art surgical techniques, where novel procedural modalities are changing the face of achalasia treatment.

3. Cutting-Edge Surgical Approaches:

Traditionally, surgery has been the mainstay of treatment for achalasia. The most effective way to alleviate symptoms and restore esophageal function is through conventional myotomy procedures. Modern clinical trials, on the other hand, have sparked a new wave of surgical innovation, with cutting-edge methods and improvements aimed at maximising the effectiveness, safety, and patient-centered results of achalasia surgical procedures.

Less invasive surgical myotomy is a significant development in the field of achalasia surgery. It uses robotic or laparoscopic assistance to perform accurate myotomies with less invasive surgery. These methods provide for the precise dissection of the esophageal musculature, addressing the underlying motor dysfunction of achalasia with improved precision and less procedure morbidity by utilising sophisticated surgical instrumentation and imaging technologies.

Comparative research and clinical trials have demonstrated the benefits of minimally invasive surgical myotomy in the treatment of achalasia, with safety and efficacy profiles that are on par with or better than those of open surgical techniques. The permanence of symptom relief and restoration of esophageal function achieved by minimally invasive surgical myotomy has been further supported by long-term follow-up data, so solidifying its position as a cornerstone of contemporary achalasia care.

The addition of minimally invasive surgical myotomy to the surgical toolkit for achalasia represents a progression toward more accurate procedures, less intrusive methods, and better patient outcomes. Through the provision of advantages such as shortened recovery times, decreased discomfort after surgery, and enhanced aesthetic outcomes, these methods reframe the surgical encounter for achalasia and promote a change in perspective towards individualised, minimally invasive procedures. To sum up, the current clinical trials for achalasia mark the beginning of a revolutionary phase in the treatment of this intricate esophageal disorder. Innovative surgical methods, sophisticated endoscopic procedures, and innovative pharmaceutical interventions are all revolutionising the field of treatment. Future achalasia therapy techniques could be individualised and multimodal, addressing patient preferences and various clinical profiles, opening up new avenues for achalasia management as long as these trials continue to provide encouraging findings and improve the therapeutic arsenal.

Genetic Research: Unraveling the DNA of Achalasia

The complex interactions between genetics and disease aetiology have long piqued the interest of researchers in the medical domain. The role of genetic variables has become increasingly relevant in the context of achalasia, a complex esophageal motility condition typified by missing peristalsis and poor relaxation of the lower esophageal sphincter (LES). This chapter aims to explore the emerging field of genetic research in achalasia and explain the ongoing efforts to identify the DNA that underlies this mysterious disorder. In order to clarify the complex relationship between genetics and the clinical symptoms of achalasia, this discourse will examine the genetic landscape of achalasia and its possible implications for disease understanding and management. An important field of study is the genetic basis of achalasia, where studies are being conducted to clarify the intricate relationship between genetic susceptibility, molecular mechanisms, and the pathophysiology of the disease. A strong amount of evidence supports the base of genetic research on achalasia, including genome-wide association studies, familial aggregation studies, and molecular studies focusing on potential genes involved in sphincter and esophageal motility. The existence of familial clustering and heritability patterns in achalasia has been repeatedly highlighted by familial aggregation studies, highlighting the possible role of genetic factors in disease vulnerability. Furthermore, genomic loci and allelic variations linked to achalasia susceptibility have been found by genome-wide association studies, providing important new information about the genetic makeup of this condition. Simultaneously, molecular studies have clarified the role of genes controlling neurotransmission, smooth muscle function, and immunological modulation in the pathogenesis of achalasia, offering a mechanistic framework for the hereditary basis of the condition.

A prominent pattern of achalasia clustering within families has been shown by familial aggregation studies, and first-degree relatives of affected individuals have been found to have a considerably greater risk of achalasia. This pattern of familial aggregation suggests that inherited genetic variants may play a role in illness susceptibility by indicating a significant genetic component in the predisposition to achalasia. Additionally, several genetic loci, such as the major histocompatibility complex (MHC) area, have been discovered by genome-wide association analysis as susceptibility loci for achalasia, highlighting the genetic complexity and heterogeneity of the disease. Interestingly, these locations include genes related to smooth muscle contraction, immunological control, and neurotrophic signalling, indicating the diverse genetic pathways linked to the pathophysiology of achalasia. Parallel to this, molecular studies have clarified the functional significance of putative genes like immune regulatory gene HLA-DQ, esophageal smooth muscle contractile protein alpha-actin (ACTA2), and cholinergic receptor muscarinic 3 (CHRM3) in the dysregulated esophageal motor function characteristic of achalasia. These findings have created a molecular framework for the genetic foundations of the disease. Even though there is strong evidence that achalasia has a genetic basis, it is important to recognise the limits and potential confounding factors that come with genetic studies. Specifically, a thorough understanding of gene-environment interactions is required due to the intricate interplay between genetic predisposition and environmental factors in the pathogenesis of achalasia. Furthermore, the complex nature of genetic vulnerability is highlighted by the genetic heterogeneity and allelic variety seen in achalasia, which calls for thorough replication studies and functional characterisation of genetic variations to determine their pathogenic relevance. Aims are being made to clarify the interaction of genetic and environmental elements in disease aetiology in response to the possible shortcomings of genetic research in achalasia. The dynamic interplay between genetic predisposition and environmental effects in achalasia susceptibility is set to be uncovered by collaborative projects that integrate multi-omic analysis, environmental exposure assessments, and gene-environment interaction investigations. Furthermore, by bridging the gap between genetic correlations and disease pathophysiology, functional characterisation studies and in vitro modelling of genetic variations provide avenues to delineate the mechanistic consequences of genetic abnormalities in esophageal motor dysfunction. The convergence of data from genome-wide association studies, familial aggregation studies, and molecular investigations highlights the complicated genetic basis of achalasia and emphasises the need for thorough genetic investigations to fully understand the disorder's complex pathophysiology. Large-scale genetic studies and meta-analyses have also been made possible by cooperative international consortia and biobanking initiatives. These efforts have allowed for the discovery of novel genetic determinants and pathways linked to the development of achalasia and susceptibility to the disease. In summary, the rapidly developing field of genetic research in achalasia represents a revolutionary frontier in our knowledge of and ability to treat this complex esophageal condition. The complex genetic architecture of achalasia is highlighted by the convincing data from genome-wide association studies, familial aggregation studies, and molecular research, which signals a paradigm change toward individualised, genetics-informed approaches to illness management. The field of achalasia management could undergo a significant transformation with the introduction of targeted therapies based on individual genetic profiles. This would usher in a new era of genetically informed precision care for patients suffering from this difficult condition, as genetic research continues to uncover the DNA foundations of achalasia.

A prominent pattern of achalasia clustering within families has been shown by familial aggregation studies, and first-degree relatives of affected individuals have been found to have a considerably greater risk of achalasia. This pattern of familial aggregation suggests that inherited genetic variants may play a role in illness susceptibility by indicating a significant genetic component in the predisposition to achalasia. Additionally, several genetic loci, such as the major histocompatibility complex (MHC) area, have been discovered by genome-wide association analysis as susceptibility loci for achalasia, highlighting the genetic complexity and heterogeneity of the disease. Interestingly, these locations include genes related to smooth muscle contraction, immunological control, and neurotrophic signalling, indicating the diverse genetic pathways linked to the pathophysiology of achalasia. Parallel to this, molecular studies have clarified the functional significance of putative genes like immune regulatory gene HLA-DQ, esophageal smooth muscle contractile protein alpha-actin (ACTA2), and cholinergic receptor muscarinic 3 (CHRM3) in the dysregulated esophageal motor function characteristic of achalasia. These findings have created a molecular framework for the genetic foundations of the disease. Even though there is strong evidence that achalasia has a genetic basis, it is important to recognise the limits and potential confounding factors that come with genetic studies. Specifically, a thorough understanding of gene-environment interactions is required due to the intricate interplay between genetic predisposition and environmental factors in the pathogenesis of achalasia. Furthermore, the complex nature of genetic vulnerability is highlighted by the genetic heterogeneity and allelic variety seen in achalasia, which calls for thorough replication studies and functional characterisation of genetic variations to determine their pathogenic relevance. Aims are being made to clarify the interaction of genetic and environmental elements in disease aetiology in response to the possible shortcomings of genetic research in achalasia. The dynamic interplay between genetic predisposition and environmental effects in achalasia susceptibility is set to be uncovered by collaborative projects that integrate multi-omic analysis, environmental exposure assessments, and gene-environment interaction investigations. Furthermore, by bridging the gap between genetic correlations and disease pathophysiology, functional characterisation studies and in vitro modelling of genetic variations provide avenues to delineate the mechanistic consequences of genetic abnormalities in esophageal motor dysfunction. The convergence of data from genome-wide association studies, familial aggregation studies, and molecular investigations highlights the complicated genetic basis of achalasia and emphasises the need for thorough genetic investigations to fully understand the disorder's complex pathophysiology. Large-scale genetic studies and meta-analyses have also been made possible by cooperative international consortia and biobanking initiatives. These efforts have allowed for the discovery of novel genetic determinants and pathways linked to the development of achalasia and susceptibility to the disease. In summary, the rapidly developing field of genetic research in achalasia represents a revolutionary frontier in our knowledge of and ability to treat this complex esophageal condition. The complex genetic architecture of achalasia is highlighted by the convincing data from genome-wide association studies, familial aggregation studies, and molecular research, which signals a paradigm change toward individualised, genetics-informed approaches to illness management. The field of achalasia management could undergo a significant transformation with the introduction of targeted therapies based on individual genetic profiles. This would usher in a new era of genetically informed precision care for patients suffering from this difficult condition, as genetic research continues to uncover the DNA foundations of achalasia.

The Quest for a Cure: How Close Are We?

The long road to finding a treatment for achalasia has yielded important discoveries on the pathophysiology of this mysterious condition. But even with the amazing advancements in understanding the immunological, neurological, and genetic foundations of achalasia, finding a permanent solution is still extremely difficult. Given that science and medicine are on the verge of a breakthrough, it is critical to evaluate the state of achalasia research today and investigate the crucial question: How near are we to finding a cure for achalasia?

The main problem facing the achalasia group is that there isn't a treatment for this complex esophageal motility disorder that works for everyone. Although pharmaceutical treatments, laparoscopic Heller myotomy, and pneumatic dilation are effective symptomatic management techniques, they are not a permanent cure. The innate variability of achalasia, which includes multiple subgroups with differing esophageal motor dysfunction and clinical presentation, makes the search for a single treatment more challenging. Furthermore, the complex interactions among genetic susceptibility, immunological dysregulation, and brain dysfunction in achalasia highlight how difficult it will be to find a treatment.

The lack of a conclusive treatment for achalasia has significant consequences for affected individuals, including ongoing symptom load, reduced quality of life, and the ongoing requirement for long-term illness management. The repeated nature of dysphagia, regurgitation, and chest pain—symptoms of achalasia that cause significant physical suffering as well as psychological misery and social constraints. In addition, the dependence on palliative interventions results in significant healthcare expenses and resource use since they do not offer a permanent cure, adding to the burden of managing chronic diseases. As a result, the unfulfilled need for a curative treatment affects not just the experiences of individual patients but also the larger healthcare system.

Finding a permanent treatment for achalasia requires a multidisciplinary strategy that incorporates the emerging knowledge from immunological discoveries, genetic studies, and neurodegenerative models. The potential for a cure for achalasia appears to be enhanced by the confluence of targeted therapies, regenerative interventions, and precision medicine. A holistic approach to treatment can be envisioned by utilising the complex genetic foundations, resolving the immunological dysregulation, and addressing the neurodegenerative aspects of achalasia.

Achalasia requires a synergistic mix of immunomodulatory approaches, regenerative medicines, and genetic screening to execute a therapeutic paradigm. Precision medicine techniques, customised to each patient's unique genetic makeup, have the ability to uncover focused treatment strategies that lessen the underlying pathogenic pathways of achalasia. Furthermore, immunomodulatory techniques intended to restore immunological homeostasis in the esophageal milieu, in conjunction with regenerative therapies focusing on neuronal and muscle regeneration, may result in a treatment paradigm for achalasia.

The therapeutic paradigm that is being envisioned for achalasia has the potential to yield revolutionary results, including the complete remission of the condition, the restoration of esophageal function, and long-term symptom relief. Through the application of genetic research findings, immunological developments, and neurodegenerative models, the anticipated results of a treatment strategy include the reduction of dysphagia and regurgitation, the mitigation of esophageal dysmotility, and the restoration of esophageal peristalsis. In addition, the expected results include slowing down the course of the disease, having the possibility of a long-lasting remission, and not needing palliative care in the long run.

Although the proposed treatment paradigm offers a thorough method of tackling the complex nature of achalasia, it is crucial to recognise other options that could support the search for a permanent cure. Alternative techniques that potentially enhance the toolkit for managing achalasia include bioelectronic therapies that target brain regulation, sophisticated endoscopic interventions that provide minimally invasive approaches, and cutting-edge regenerative medicine modalities. Moreover, combining patient-centered care approaches with holistic wellness programmes, nutritional optimization, and psychosocial support can enhance the overall management of achalasia in a complementary way.

To sum up, the search for a permanent treatment for achalasia is a groundbreaking area in the field of esophageal motility disorders. At the brink of scientific discovery and therapeutic advances lies the possibility of realising a cure for achalasia through the convergence of genetic discoveries, immunological developments, and neurodegenerative paradigms. The hunt for a cure for achalasia is an unwavering undertaking that is driven by our shared dedication to reducing the impact of this mysterious condition and ushering in a new era of precision treatment for achalasia patients, even as we negotiate the complex terrain of achalasia research.

Innovations in Diagnostic Technology

In the past, esophageal motility testing, radiographic imaging, and clinical assessment have all been used to diagnose achalasia. But the search for quicker and more precise diagnostic methods has led to the investigation of cutting-edge technologies that could completely alter the field of achalasia diagnosis. In order to fill a key gap in the comprehensive management of this intricate esophageal motility problem, this chapter aims to clarify the advances in diagnostic technology that could greatly improve the accuracy, efficacy, and accessibility of achalasia diagnosis.

A paradigm shift in the diagnostic arsenal for achalasia is presented by the integration of cutting-edge diagnostic tools, including high-resolution manometry, esophageal impedance testing, and new imaging modalities. These cutting-edge technologies have the potential to improve the precision of diagnoses, facilitate the early diagnosis of diseases, and inform customised treatment plans.

As a key component of the diagnostic procedure for achalasia, high-resolution esophageal manometry (HRM) provides previously unheard-of insights into esophageal motor function. The unique pressure topography patterns identified by HRM help to distinguish between different subtypes of achalasia and offer useful prognostic data that helps choose the best course of treatment. Furthermore, the introduction of the Chicago Classification criteria has improved diagnostic consistency and clinical relevance by standardising the interpretation of HRM data.

The capacity of HRM to distinguish between the typical esophageal motor abnormalities, such as decreased lower esophageal sphincter relaxation, aperistalsis, and pan-esophageal pressurisation, highlights the critical role that HRM plays in the diagnosis of achalasia. Provocative manoeuvres like the rapid drink challenge and multiple water swallows have also been added, which has increased the diagnostic yield of HRM. This allows for the dynamic assessment of esophageal motility and makes it easier to identify subtle motor abnormalities that may not be detected by traditional diagnostic methods.

While there are unquestionably many benefits to using HRM to explain the pathognomonic features of achalasia, there are also drawbacks. These include the requirement for specialised knowledge in interpretation, a testing infrastructure that consumes a lot of resources, and difficulties in distinguishing achalasia from other esophageal motility disorders that share manometric findings. Moreover, the dynamic terrain of achalasia classification, characterised by continuous improvements in subtype definition, demands that HRM criteria be continuously validated and standardised in order to guarantee diagnostic precision and clinical significance.

Efforts should be made to improve training in the interpretation of complex manometric patterns, standardise interpretation criteria, and promote interdisciplinary collaboration between radiologists, gastroenterologists, and motility specialists in order to reduce the limitations of HRM in the context of achalasia diagnosis. Furthermore, the use of other diagnostic modalities, including sophisticated imaging techniques and esophageal impedance testing, can supplement the data obtained from HRM, providing a holistic diagnostic approach that surpasses the limitations of individual modalities.

A significant development in the diagnostic characterisation of achalasia is the introduction of esophageal high-resolution impedance manometry, which integrates the evaluation of esophageal pressure topography with the identification of bolus transit and flow dynamics. In addition to defining the motor abnormalities typical of achalasia, this integrated modality offers insights into the dynamics of bolus clearance, esophageal emptying, and the effects of decreased peristalsis on esophageal function. Additionally, a thorough evaluation of esophageal biomechanics and luminal dimensions is provided by the integration of adjunctive diagnostic techniques, such as the functional luminal imaging probe (FLIP) and esophageal 3D-imaging modalities, which improves the accuracy of diagnosis and therapeutic decision-making in achalasia.

To sum up, the development of diagnostic technologies in the field of achalasia diagnosis signals the beginning of a revolutionary period marked by improved diagnostic accuracy and customised treatment plans. Combining esophageal impedance testing, high-resolution manometry, and new imaging modalities enhances the diagnostic toolkit and gives physicians a more comprehensive picture of bolus dynamics and esophageal motor function. The promise of early disease detection, customised therapeutic interventions, and better patient outcomes looms large in the horizon as these cutting-edge technologies continue to hone our diagnostic skills, pushing the field of achalasia management toward previously unheard-of levels of accuracy and effectiveness.

Patient Advocacy and Awareness Campaigns

I am committed to advancing holistic healthcare and wellbeing as a medical doctor and health and wellness coach. In order to effectively treat patients with achalasia, I use a multidisciplinary team approach that incorporates lifestyle changes, dietary planning, counselling, psychology, self-care practises, and coping mechanisms. We will examine the vital role that public awareness campaigns and patient advocacy play in advancing achalasia patient care and research in this chapter.

Compiling a background of important information about the setting and environment for the case study is essential to comprehending the influence of awareness and advocacy efforts in the field of achalasia management. Achalasia is a condition marked by decreased esophageal motility. Patients may have dysphagia, regurgitation, chest pain, and weight loss. The condition's infrequency and complexity frequently result in improper treatment and delayed diagnosis, which exacerbates the emotional and physical toll that sufferers and their families must bear. In light of this, it is imperative that strong advocacy and awareness campaigns be launched in order to advance research, raise diagnostic awareness, and raise the standard of treatment for people with achalasia.

It is essential to provide pertinent background information to the main characters or entities in the case study in order to comprehend the dynamics of advocacy and awareness campaigns within the framework of managing achalasia. Advocates for patients, medical professionals, researchers, and legislators are the primary participants in the advocacy and awareness space for achalasia. Patient advocacy organisations play a crucial role in amplifying patient voices, cultivating community support, and championing research funding and legislative reforms.

Examples of these organisations are the Achalasia Foundation and the International Foundation for Gastrointestinal Disorders. Together, researchers and healthcare professionals are essential in advancing patient-centered care pathways, encouraging early diagnosis, and spreading accurate information. Through thoughtful advocacy and well-planned awareness campaigns, policymakers, who have the power to affect healthcare policies and budget allocation, are another important factor in determining how achalasia management is shaped in the field.

Understanding the necessity of advocacy and awareness activities in the field of achalasia management is made easier by clearly identifying the central problem or difficulty of the case study. The complex issues include a lack of awareness of the symptoms of achalasia, delayed diagnosis, few available treatments, and the psychological effects on the patients. Additionally, the stigma associated with achalasia contributes to the marginalisation of patients and makes it more difficult to provide funds for specialist care and research. In order to overcome these obstacles, a concentrated effort must be made to support patient-centered treatment, encourage early diagnosis, and cultivate a helpful ecosystem that equips patients and healthcare professionals with reliable data and tools.

Giving a detailed account of the particular approaches or techniques employed to tackle the problem in the case study sheds light on the complex nature of advocacy and awareness campaigns in the management of achalasia. The promotion of achalasia awareness through informational campaigns, support networks, and social media platforms is included in advocacy initiatives. The aforementioned measures are designed to de-stigmatize the ailment, enable patients to obtain prompt medical attention, and encourage healthcare providers to embrace patient-centered methodologies. Advocacy groups also work with scientists and legislators to push for more financing for studies on achalasia, clinical trials for new treatments, and the creation of clinical guidelines emphasising patient-centered care and holistic therapy.

When data is available, highlighting the results and effects of the chosen strategy provides a concrete example of the effectiveness of advocacy and awareness raising in the management of achalasia. Positive effects include a greater sense of community and support for patients and their families, a decrease in diagnostic delays due to increased public knowledge improving the recognition of achalasia symptoms. Additionally, cutting-edge research on novel treatment modalities, lifestyle modifications, and psychosocial support models catered to the particular requirements of achalasia patients has been sparked by advocacy-driven research funding. All of these results demonstrate the real influence that advocacy and awareness efforts have on bringing about revolutionary shifts in the field of achalasia management.

A comprehensive evaluation of the complex nature of advocacy and awareness campaigns in achalasia management is made possible by providing thoughts and views on the case study's lessons and possible drawbacks. In order to bring about significant change, the case study emphasises the critical role that patient advocacy plays in shaping healthcare legislation, encouraging research partnerships, and elevating patient voices. Potential objections, however, can centre on the necessity of advocacy initiatives maintaining momentum, the fair allocation of resources, and the inclusion of various patient viewpoints in the development of awareness campaigns and care routes. Considering these subtleties highlights the need for advocacy and awareness campaigns to constantly evolve and improve in order to maintain their relevance and long-term influence in the management of achalasia.

For example, infographics that illustrate how advocacy and awareness efforts affect patient outcomes, diagnosis times, and research advances can be used to improve comprehension of the case study.

Testimonials from patients, medical experts, and researchers demonstrating the game-changing impact of advocacy and awareness campaigns in the field of achalasia management could also be included as visual aids.

Connecting the case study's specifics to the major issue or underlying themes emphasises how advocacy and awareness campaigns are part of the larger storey of managing achalasia. The case study is in line with the underlying requirement to support early diagnosis, encourage patient-centered care, and propel research advancements that raise the bar for patients with achalasia. The case study also emphasises how crucial advocacy is in building an inclusive ecosystem, demythologizing misunderstandings, and inspiring community support that enables patients to face achalasia head-on and make wise decisions.

In order to promote further involvement, it is important to leave the reader with a question or a connected thought. This involves provoking contemplation on our shared duty for spearheading advocacy and awareness campaigns that aim to change the face of achalasia management. How can a range of stakeholders, such as patients, healthcare professionals, researchers, and legislators, work together to effectively utilise advocacy and awareness campaigns in order to promote a more understanding, just, and encouraging framework for the treatment of achalasia?

The case study concludes by highlighting the paradigm-shifting impact of advocacy and awareness initiatives in the management of achalasia. These programmes, which have raised public awareness, encouraged research collaborations, and amplified patient voices, have sparked a paradigm shift in the support of prompt diagnosis, patient-centered care, and scientific discoveries that improve the quality of life for patients with achalasia. The ongoing dedication to advocacy and awareness campaigns is essential to promoting long-lasting, patient-centered improvements that support the philosophy of holistic wellbeing and empowerment for achalasia patients and their families as we negotiate the changing terrain of achalasia therapy.

The Role of Artificial Intelligence in Achalasia

It is becoming more and more clear as we explore the complex world of managing achalasia that adopting cutting-edge strategies is essential to improving patient outcomes, treatment efficacy, and diagnostic accuracy. An innovative approach that has great potential to transform the management of achalasia is the application of artificial intelligence (AI) to the understanding, diagnosis, and treatment of this intricate esophageal motility condition.

Artificial intelligence, or AI for short, is the term used to describe how computers, especially computer systems, may mimic human intelligence processes. Self-correction, reasoning, and learning are some of these processes. Potential AI applications in achalasia management have the potential to completely change the way that care is provided by improving the precision of diagnosis, refining treatment plans, and enabling individualised patient care paths. The objective of this chapter is to clarify the revolutionary function of artificial intelligence (AI) in the all-encompassing management of achalasia, including its influence on patient-centered care, therapy optimization, and diagnostic techniques.

Using sophisticated computer algorithms, machine learning models, and data analytics, the integration of artificial intelligence in achalasia management takes a multipronged approach to interpreting intricate patterns found in patient data, diagnostic imaging results, and treatment outcomes. The ability of AI-driven diagnostic tools to precisely assess esophageal motility patterns allows for the early identification of achalasia and its distinction from other esophageal illnesses. Predictive models driven by AI can also clarify customised therapy responses, improving the therapeutic strategy for every patient according to their particular physiological and clinical characteristics.

To illustrate how AI can revolutionise the treatment of achalasia, imagine a patient who presents with unusual symptoms that defy standard diagnostic criteria. Clinicians can identify small motility anomalies typical of achalasia by applying AI-driven pattern recognition algorithms to high-resolution esophageal manometry data. This allows for a prompt diagnosis and customised treatments. AI-enabled risk assessment algorithms can also forecast a patient's propensity to respond to various therapy modalities, which helps doctors create individualised treatment plans that maximise patient outcomes and reduce procedural risks.

Diverse viewpoints are fostered by the incorporation of AI in achalasia management, which captures the cooperative synergy between clinicians, patient advocates, and computational experts. From a computational perspective, AI algorithms are always improving due to iterative learning from large datasets, which helps them become more accurate at diagnosis and prognosis with every interaction. In turn, clinicians use AI-driven insights to traverse the complexities of managing achalasia and use predictive analytics to customise treatment plans that fit the individual clinical trajectory of each patient. In order to ensure that these technologies emphasise patient autonomy, data privacy, and fair access to AI-driven diagnostic and therapeutic advancements, patient advocates urge the ethical integration of AI.

Clinical studies highlighting the increased diagnosis accuracy of AI-driven esophageal motility study over traditional approaches provide strong empirical support for the inclusion of AI in achalasia care. Moreover, AI-powered risk stratification models have shown remarkably accurate in forecasting treatment results, assisting physicians in fine-tuning their approach and improving patient outcomes. All of these developments demonstrate the real-world influence of AI on enhancing the diagnostic and treatment tools available for managing achalasia.

Terms like machine learning, deep learning, and neural networks may be used often in the context of artificial intelligence. The ability of computer systems to automatically pick up new skills and improve from past experiences without explicit programming is known as machine learning. Deep learning is a branch of machine learning that focuses on teaching artificial neural networks to identify complicated patterns in datasets so that complex characteristics can be extracted for prognostic and diagnostic purposes. Deep learning algorithms are based on neural networks, which are modelled after the linked neuron structure of the human brain. This allows for the extraction of subtle patterns from physiological and medical imaging data.

To sum up, the incorporation of artificial intelligence into the management of achalasia signals the beginning of a revolutionary period marked by patient-centered care, tailored treatment optimization, and precise diagnosis. AI enables physicians to decipher the complicated intricacies of achalasia, promoting early diagnosis, customised treatment plans, and improved patient outcomes. It does this by utilising sophisticated computer algorithms and machine learning models. AI's ethical incorporation into the therapy of achalasia promises to improve care standards and spark a paradigm change in the comprehensive treatment of this puzzling esophageal motility condition as it develops.

We will go into more detail on the specific uses of AI in achalasia management in the upcoming chapters, explaining how patient advocacy, clinical practise, and computational advances interact to change the face of achalasia care. We seek to provide clinicians, researchers, and patient advocates with a nuanced understanding of the transformative potential of artificial intelligence in navigating the complexities of achalasia management through a thorough investigation of AI-driven diagnostic tools, predictive modelling, and therapeutic optimization.

Global Collaboration in Achalasia Research

Welcome to "The Achalasia Mastery Bible: Your Complete Achalasia Management Blueprint." I boldly promise you, the reader, that after reading this comprehensive guide, you will have a complete understanding of achalasia, its management, and how to confidently and empowered traverse the complexity of this difficult condition.

As a physician and health and wellness advisor, I recognise the value of a comprehensive approach to treatment. This book combines my knowledge with the collective experience of a wide range of professionals in the wellness and health sectors. I will give you a complete toolkit to effectively manage achalasia through evidence-based approaches, lifestyle changes, customised food and diet planning, counselling and psychology techniques, and a variety of self-care and coping mechanisms.

You might be sceptical about the efficacy of treating a disorder as complicated as achalasia. You may be confident that this book is more than just a compilation of general information. This resource has been painstakingly created, utilising the most recent findings, clinical knowledge, and the combined experiences of patients and caregivers. It has been demonstrated that the methods described in these pages can significantly enhance the quality of life for people who suffer achalasia.

Imagine a life free from the overwhelming weight of achalasia's problems. Imagine yourself in the future, armed with the information and resources necessary to manage your disease with resilience and self-assurance. This book serves as your road map for such change, taking you step-by-step through the process of managing achalasia holistically.

This book's substance is transformative rather than merely educational. You will be able to manage achalasia more skillfully and regain control over your health by assimilating the techniques and knowledge shared here. Despite the difficulties of achalasia, you can have a better, more satisfying life if you read this book and put its teachings into practise.

I encourage you to approach the upcoming chapters with an open mind and a readiness to embrace change as we set off on this life-changing trip together. Your commitment to this process will be crucial in enabling the possibility of a more promising and self-assured future despite achalasia.

www.ingramcontent.com/pod-product-compliance
Ingram Content Group UK Ltd.
Pitfield, Milton Keynes, MK11 3LW, UK
UKHW020731280125
4322UKWH00046B/538